DEATH BY DECEPTION

Unmasking Heart Failure

DICK QUINN, SHANNON QUINN,
COLIN QUINN AND AL WATSON

Cover Design: **Marysarah Quinn**

Design & Typography: **JEZAC Type & Design**

Illustrations by:
Karen Berry, Karla Caspari and Kathy Vaneps

WITH SPECIAL THANKS TO TOM QUINN, ROY UPTON, JAMES GREEN, DAVID HOFFMANN, DANIEL MOWREY; AND DR. JOHN CHRISTOPHER WHO TAUGHT THE "LADY OF THE LAKE" THE SECRETS OF CAYENNE PEPPER SO LONG AGO.

"Death by Deception: Unmasking Heart Failure"
© Copyright 1996 by Shannon Quinn, Dick Quinn,
Colin Quinn and Al Watson

1st printing July 1996

ISBN 0-9653346-0-0 $12.95 U.S.

R.F. QUINN PUBLISHING CO.
P.O. Box 17100 • Minneapolis, MN 55417
(800) 283-3998

NOTE TO THE READER:
While diet, herbs and supplements can play an important role in preventing or alleviating degenerative conditions like congestive heart failure (CHF), it should be done under the supervision of a health care professional. It is advisable to seek professional medical care for the diagnosis and treatment of serious conditions like CHF and its causes.

DEDICATED
TO THE
MEMORY OF
DICK QUINN

ABOUT THE AUTHORS

DICK QUINN, author of the international best-seller *Left For Dead*, was a professional writer and a self taught herbalist. *Left for Dead* is the true story of how Cayenne Pepper and other herbs saved Quinn's life after his coronary bypass surgery failed.

    Death by Deception: Unmasking Heart Failure is the sequel to *Left for Dead* and Dick Quinn's final work. In "A Letter to Sally" and Part I of "A Case of Heart Failure," Quinn tells of his personal experience with a deadly condition that awaits unsuspecting victims of heart disease - congestive heart failure.

SHANNON QUINN takes up the story of Dick Quinn's courageous fight against heart failure from a daughter's perspective in Part II of *A Case of Heart Failure*. A journalist for over a decade, Shannon was a co-author of *Left For Dead*. She wrote the section on the healing power of herbs for the heart.

    In the chapter "Medicines in the Meadow," Shannon focuses on herbs for the prevention and treatment of congestive heart failure. "Medicines of the Meadow" features cardiac formulas created by renowned herbalists and a detailed description of each of the herbs used to fight heart failure.

COLIN QUINN'S two-part medical section, "Anatomy of a Killer" and "Medical Approaches to Heart Failure," explains the complexities of congestive heart failure. He explores the causes, symptoms and treatments of the debilitating condition.

    Colin, who holds a degree in English from the University of Minnesota, wrote the medical section in *Left for Dead*. He and his wife Julie, a registered nurse, began researching heart failure after Dick Quinn was diagnosed in December 1994.

AL WATSON achieved success using food as medicine to help his long-time friend Dick Quinn and in the process created the first diet for heart failure. Watson, who owned a health store for many years, discusses those healing foods and the pathways to heart failure in his section titled "Fueling the Fight Against Heart Failure."

    Watson holds a degree in history and now operates an herbal supplement company in Sebeka, Minnesota.

CONTENTS

SECTION IV – *by Al Watson*

FUELING THE FIGHT AGAINST HEART FAILURE

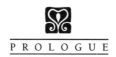

A LETTER TO SALLY

Letter from Dick Quinn to his sister Sally Hansen
written Jan. 31, 1995 – nearly two months after doctors
predicted he would not live through the night.

Hi Sal,

I hope this finds you and yours in good health and prospering. I seem to be getting slowly, slowly better.

I'm still taking a ton of stuff – about 91 pills a day at the moment. I get up every day feeling fine, then take this vomitous soup of vitamins, hormones, minerals, herbs and drugs which makes me sick for most of the day. I spend all day recovering and get a few things done in the evening. Not much of a life, but I have to do it until next summer.

I'm now waiting for a new substance from Germany which is supposed to neutralize the acidity in my left ventricle. The acidity is what kills you, so it's kind of important to get rid of it.

This is actually a rather ghastly disorder. It's like being suffocated or drowning. Your lungs fill with fluid, your heart gets big (mine was described as "enormous") and speeds up (mine hit 300 beats per minute – like a hummingbird), and only pumps half the blood it should, so you get half the oxygen you need. Then it breaks.

My heart made it through because of the Cayenne and other herbs I take, in my opinion. I guess I passed the breaking point by quite a way. They all pronounced me dead at the hospital, but I actually felt fine.

The problem with this congestive heart failure is that it's so fast. I didn't realize anything was wrong one day, and the next I couldn't walk 10 feet without resting. I was suddenly gaining 3 pounds a day in water. When I finally got "drained," I lost about 15 pounds in six hours. It was quite spectacular.

I have just started to write a book about it – calling it "Not Dead Yet." It's a good way to spend time at home and get my mind off this health thing – as well as helping people who get this.

I just read that congestive heart failure is the fastest growing coronary disorder. Very trendy. Nearly everybody who gets it dies, but I'm dodging the bullet and I want to tell everyone how I did it. I'm not going to be doing it again.

There are no books on it and very little is known. Normally, you just take the drugs until they do a heart transplant, which is bullshit. I'm going to heal my heart.

The drugs all destroy your quality of life and eventually kill you. That's why everybody who gets it dies – but not me. I'm going to get healthy again with the help of my Italian-Jewish-Hindu doctor, a guy in Germany and a few other people including myself.

My doctor is an M.D. who learned medicine and herbalism in Europe and was a close friend of Linus Pauling, the vitamin C guy. He knows all the famous alternative M.D.s and has me taking all sorts of hormones.

I'm going to spend the spring and early summer getting well, publish a damned good book about it and take the Queen Elizabeth II to Europe, where I'm going to spend part of August and all of September bumming around.

As for now, it did stop raining and it's going to be 83 today. Why worry?

Take care of yourself and yours – I'll be in touch.

Dick Quinn never made it to Europe. Seven months after this letter was written, he died of a ruptured aortic aneurysm. His ashes were scattered over County Clare, Ireland in keeping with his final wishes.

Had we known then what we learned over the course of his illness, he'd still be alive today showing off photographs of his vacation aboard the QE II.

We finished the book he started in the hope that others would then be able to complete the recovery he began.

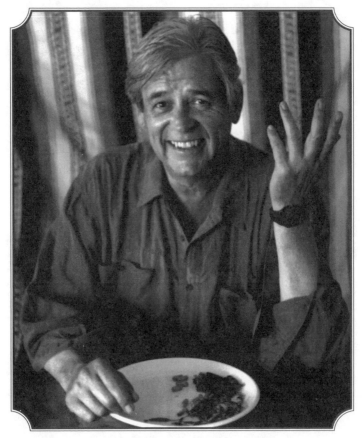

DICK MIXES A FEW CAYENNE CAPS BY HAND IN THE LIVING ROOM OF HIS MINNEAPOLIS APARTMENT.

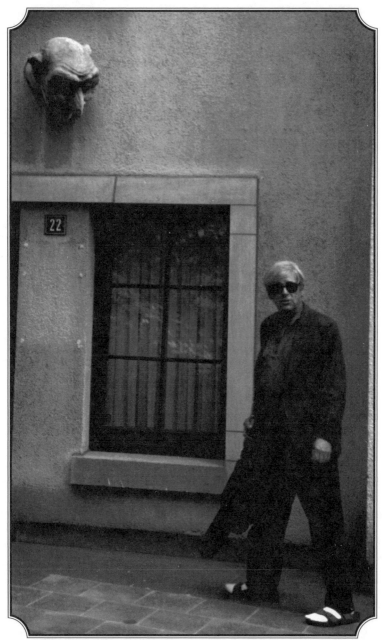

DICK ENCOUNTERS A GARGOYLE ON THE STREETS OF LUXEMBOURG.
CAYENNE FUELED HIS 1993 TRIP TO EUROPE TO PROMOTE
"LEFT FOR DEAD" AT THE FRANKFURT INTERNATIONAL BOOK FAIR.

A CASE OF HEART FAILURE

*Often the test of courage is not to die,
but to live.*

-COUNT VITTORIO ALFIERI

W hen my father discovered he had congestive heart failure, he immediately set to work on a sequel to "Left for Dead" his best-selling book on natural remedies for heart disease. He was determined that others would once again benefit from his daring experiments on himself.

My father's soul was brave but his heart was weak. He was unable to do more than write the few pages that make up Part I of this section of the book. I have taken up where he left off in the hope that this very special case history, with all its triumphs and misadventures, could help others avoid such a loss.

– Shannon Quinn

PART ONE

I knew something was wrong when I tried to walk up the hill to the post office and had to stop and rest on the curb twice in the first block.

I was strangely out of breath. It was very unpleasant; I don't remember ever feeling that way before. Fortunately, a friend came by in his truck and gave me a ride up the hill. I don't think I could have made it on my own.

The next day, I tried to walk again, but it was even worse. I had to stop after walking only 25 feet uphill. When I had to stop the second time, I gave up and went home.

I had always walked at least a mile a day, but then I injured my back on a trip to Canada. For two months after that, I couldn't walk, so my daily exercise ended.

I attributed my extreme short-windedness to "being out of shape" from lack of exercise. I had never been this out of shape. I had never been unable to breathe as I was now. It was a terrible claustrophobic feeling. Now I knew what suffocation must be like.

A few days later, I flew to Orlando for a convention. It was an early morning flight so I took a 4 a.m. shuttle to the airport and got no sleep at all that night. Canada had been a particularly difficult trip and I hadn't yet recovered from it.

On arrival in Orlando, I checked into a hotel and went to bed early. I awoke about two hours later, gasping for air in great gulps. I don't think I ever breathed so deeply, yet I couldn't get enough air into my lungs to offset the terrible feeling of suffocation.

It was especially difficult to breathe when I lay down, so I sat up the rest of the night.

I was in Orlando for seven busy days and it was like that every night. I never got more than two hours sleep. After hours of sitting up, exhausted, I would fall asleep only to be awakened with a start an instant later.

It became a nightmare. I began to imagine that an evil faceless person was trying to suffocate me whenever I relaxed my guard.

I couldn't breath but I didn't know why. Probably congestion in my lungs, I thought naively.

Exhausted, I returned from Orlando with chest pains I

thought were caused when my violent gasping breaths bruised my lungs.

I had been home about two days when my daughter Shannon called. She had been speaking with my son Foley and my daughter Kelly. They had all heard my breathing and were concerned.

"I have an appointment with my doctor this afternoon," Shannon said. "I'd like you to come along.

"He's a nice guy," she added reassuringly. "Holistic."

I hadn't seen an M.D. in 16 years – not since I took over my own health care when my coronary bypass failed and I was left for dead.

I hadn't had a good night's sleep in weeks and now I was gaining weight. Water weight, I suppose. It seemed something should be done.

It took two rest stops to make it to the door of the doctor's office – a distance of about 10 feet. They took me in right away – no time to peruse the magazines in the waiting room.

"How's the blood pressure doctor?" I asked. He looked at me ominously, but said nothing. "Kind of high huh?"

"Yeah," he smiled sardonically, "kind of high. 210 over 180."

The nurse untangled the wires and hooked me up to the electrocardiogram machine. It soon began to print out its little strips of data.

The little lines on the first couple of printouts looked normal enough. They reminded me of seismographs from an earth monitoring machine. No quakes so far. Then came one that was different. The little lines were so close together they made one broad slash across the sheet, like a wide black marker.

The doctor studied the printout, holding it to the light, trying to count the little lines but they were so closely bunched together they blended into one. He wasn't smiling anymore.

"The upper chamber of your heart is beating at 300 per minute, the lower at about 240 – it's hard to tell exactly," he said with a look of absolute consternation. "I've never seen anything like this. You have to get into the hospital at once."

"The hospital?"

It was inconceivable. I hadn't been in a hospital for 16

years – not since my heart attack and bypass. People die in hospitals. They kill you there; they treat you to death.

"Are you a member of a health group?" he continued earnestly, not noticing my dismay. "You could get in line for a heart transplant and get a pacemaker until we find a heart."

"Doctor, I have a heart," I said. "I want to heal the one I have."

He seemed puzzled by my reference to healing. "I have no insurance at all, but even if I did, there will be no transplant, there will be no pacemaker, there will be no heart surgery of any sort. If it's a choice between dying and surgery, I'll die."

"I just can't be responsible," he said, exasperated. "You don't understand. This is serious. Anything could happen. I've never seen anyone with readings this high."

"You mean I could die – that's why I should get into the hospital?" He still thought I just didn't understand.

"You have to get into the hospital at once," he said. "Do you have chest pain? Are you dizzy, sick?"

"Nothing like that. I feel fine – I just can't breathe, so I can't walk more than 10 feet without sitting down."

"You could die at any time. I'm surprised to see you sitting there. Your heart should have stopped already – it just can't go on beating at that rate. You shouldn't go anywhere. I really can't let you leave. I can't take the responsibility."

"Look doctor, with all due respect, most people die in the hospital. It's the most dangerous place you can be. And while I don't want to die, death is nothing new to me," I said gently.

"I don't want to appear glib, doctor. You've explained the risk and I believe you. I agree that death is damned serious – it really is the end of the world. But I've been staring it in the face since I had a heart attack in 1978, so it's nothing I haven't dealt with before."

Neither he nor my daughter Shannon interfered. They respected my right to make my own decisions about my life.

"You have congestive heart failure," he said.

"And my heart is enlarged I suppose . . ." I said.

"It's enormous."

"OK. I know what I'm up against and I have to do what I think is most likely to save my life. I have to make that decision because I'm doing the dying.

"I've heard what you said, I respect your judgment and I feel your concern is genuine, but I think it's best for me to go home and spend the weekend tending to this in my own way and then come back to see you Monday."

He looked at me skeptically, sure I'd be dead before Monday.

"I have my own stuff to take," I continued. "Herbs and things. Don't worry though – I'll take full responsibility. If you'll feel better, just write a release and I'll sign it."

He wrote the release, putting the 911 emergency number on the top. "Be sure to call this if anything happens," he cautioned, directing his remark to Shannon in a tone that suggested something surely would.

"Don't worry doctor, I'll be fine."

They got me into a wheelchair and helped Shannon wheel me out to the car. "See you Monday doctor," I said. I could see he was really concerned about me – nothing phony like I've experienced with so many medical professionals.

I didn't like to worry him so, but I had to do what I felt was best for me, what was safest. I felt it was safest to go home, where I could take my Cayenne to keep my heart pumping and Dandelion leaf to safely get rid of the water that was now building up at the rate of three pounds per day and suffocating me. I was drowning.

I had congestive heart failure. You die from that. The water buildup makes your heart run so fast it breaks.

They give you Digitalis to slow down your heart and keep it pumping. It's a poison derived from the herb Foxglove.

It might keep you pumping for awhile but it eventually kills you because it's a cumulative drug. What begins as a safe dose eventually becomes a fatal overdose. I knew all about it. I also knew that Lily of the Valley is safer.

They also give you Lasix – a terrible diuretic that gets rid of the water build-up but also takes out your minerals so your heartbeat becomes erratic and that kills you.

Digitalis and Lasix. You can't win with them. I knew I might have to resort to them eventually, but I wanted to try my own stuff first.

Part Two

Sitting in his office one day, alone in the house, my father made a deadly decision. Like choosing to ski the closed trail, going for a midnight swim alone or stepping on a tightrope without a safety net, my father began a dangerous secret experiment with his medication.

Almost a year later, I stumbled on the plan he had written down that day. Black letters screamed off the white paper: "Taking Lanoxin .25 mg since 12-14-94. Reduce to 1/2 tablet daily from 1-23 to 1-26, 1/4 tablet daily 1-27 to 1-29, then discontinue use. Tell no one."

Oh, there is nothing I would not give to go back in time and change those last three fatal words. His secret cost him dearly. He suffered a setback so severe, he would never fully recover.

My father had always disdained drugs like Lanoxin (Digitalis) because of such nasty side-effects as sudden death. He'd done enough research on herbs to know Digitalis, which comes from the Foxglove plant, is a cumulative poison. Over time, it builds up to a toxic level in your blood stream and can kill you.

With Digitalis, you're damned if you do, damned if you don't. If you don't take enough of it, you can get worse and die. If you take it too long you can also get worse and die. For heart failure as advanced as my father's, Digitalis was a lifeline. Alone in his den that day, he decided to cut the cord.

As it turns out, he didn't have to do anything that drastic. He didn't realize it then but he was already in the process of cutting back on Digitalis naturally. Over time, the Hawthorn he was taking would enhance the action of Digitalis, lowering the necessary dosage and reducing the chances of toxic accumulation.

My father dropped his "doctor du jour" and the Digitalis at about the same time. The doctor had tried to discourage him from his plan, emphasizing how important the drug was in the later stages of congestive heart failure.

There were other types of doctors who would have supported my father's decision to substitute his homemade heart formula with Lily of the Valley, a powerful herbal cardiac stimulant. He didn't seek that critical second opinion. As a successful self-taught herbalist, he figured he could do it himself and adjust the dosage as he went along – but his condition was too delicate.

Dad's fatal error was not his decision to get off the drug but how he handled it. The danger of getting off any powerful drug is that the body has learned to rely on it so that any change can be a shock to the system. A highly trained herbalist or naturopathic doctor could have safely weaned my father off Digitalis by gradually substituting herbs like Lily of the Valley and Cactus Grandiflorus, as is commonly done in Europe.

You can be independent without going it alone. Leave your medical options open and choose which you want to use. As the saying goes, "Knowledge is power." Knowing what all the alternatives are gives you true control of your own health care. You're still in the driver's seat, you're just asking for directions so you don't get lost. For example, you don't have to believe in taking blood pressure medication to go get your blood pressure checked.

Instead of seeking professional help, my father was flying blind. While his Digitalis levels had been carefully monitored by his doctors, he had no idea if he was taking too much or too little Lily of the Valley. He was only guessing how much of the herb it would take to make up for the Digitalis he'd be losing.

As the level of Digitalis ebbed, my father got noticeably weaker and more breathless. At first he slept all day but soon his breathing became more labored and he couldn't sleep at all for fear of suffocation. The fluid started coming back, stiffening his feet, ankles and calves. As his heart began to struggle without the support of the Digitalis, his blood pressure crept higher.

As my father's condition began to worsen, he got a call from his friend Canadian author Byrun Tylor. Tylor had been diagnosed with severe congestive heart failure four months earlier and faxed regular "guinea pig" progress reports to my father.

That day was a bad one for Byrun as reflected in Father's journal entry: "Can't get his shoes on. He's afraid to use sleeping pills because he might not wake up."

Byrun told my father he was going to call a friend of theirs in Germany who knew of a European heart medication that might help them both. Dr. Siegfried Rilling, known as "the father of ozone therapy," gave Byrun Strodival, a heart drug derived from the African herb Strophanthus.

Strodival has been used in Germany for decades to treat heart failure. It reduces acidosis in the left ventricle that "suffocates" the heart muscle. The effect of the drug on Byrun, who also had cancer, was remarkable. Within hours of his first dose, he was on the phone to Southern California – back to his irrepressible gregarious self.

While Byrun was rebounding, my father's condition was deteriorating. His breathing was labored even at rest. No longer able to use the computer, work on his new book about congestive heart failure was suspended.

Finally, he was forced to admit to us that he had been off Digitalis for several days. To get back on track, a friend recommended he see a doctor who specialized in chelation. Chelation therapy uses intravenous injections of a manmade amino acid to remove toxic metals from the body. It has been used to treat coronary artery disease, blood clots and arrhythmia with remarkable results.

The new doctor did an extensive blood analysis, checking levels of essential minerals, hormones and other critical chemicals and confirmed that both his digoxin (Digitalis) and calcium levels were critically low. His digoxin level was down to one-tenth of what it should have been.

While digoxin stimulates his heart, calcium regulates heart rhythm. Too much calcium can cause the heart to race. Too little can cause it to beat too slow. Dad's calcium level was low and his glucose level was high. High glucose levels can lead to heart disease.

With the levels of calcium and digoxin dangerously low, the doctors said there was a crisis situation in his left ventricle. His ejection fraction was now only 19 percent – down from 40 percent in December. An ejection fraction measures the amount of blood entering the heart chambers and how much is being pumped out or "ejected." A normal ejection fraction is about 60 percent and anything below 20 is considered "crisis stage."

The doctors sent Dad home with prescriptions for a

calcium supplement and Digitalis. His condition was deemed too precarious to try chelation therapy.

Worried he'd gone too far, my father turned his attention to the Strodival that helped his friend Byrun. He hoped that the German drug would help him recover the ground he had lost by going off Digitalis. He wrote Dr. Rilling asking him to send some right away.

Unfortunately, the German doctor had problems of his own. Grieving over his wife's recent death, Rilling was in strict mourning communicating with no one save his son.

Loath to disturb the doctor, my father tried contacting Rilling's pharmacy in Stuttgart but was blocked by the language barrier. His only alternative seemed to be to wait for Dr. Rilling to come out of mourning.

Unable to sleep more than a couple of hours a night, my father woke one morning to find the fluid around his ankles was worse than ever despite the new doses of Digitalis. Constantly gasping for his next breath, the fatigue was crushing both physically and emotionally. He began to fear he wouldn't survive to celebrate his 59th Birthday which was only two days away.

The day before his birthday, like a gift from the Gods, he received a dozen "hits" of Strodival in the mail from his buddy Byrun. On Feb. 5, 1995, less than 24 hours after he took his first dose of the German drug, Dad celebrated his 59th birthday with a brunch at the Tropicana Bar and Grill – his favorite hang-out.

Sitting at the head of the table filled with family and friends, he munched on omelets and strawberry waffles and talked about plans for his birthday year – the new book, a trip to Europe and a return to "normal" life where he could walk without wheezing, sleep without nightmares and laugh at death once again. We, who had been so worried, were now filled with hope.

With only a few precious pills left, he laid low waiting for Rilling's shipment to arrive. Resting most of the day, he conserved as best he could and watched for the package Rilling said he sent two weeks earlier. But as the days passed, he grew weaker and more desperate.

He took the last Strodival on Sunday Feb. 12 – exactly a week after his jubilant birthday celebration – but the effect was far less dramatic than the first. "Didn't hit hard," he wrote in a shaky scrawl. "Still weak."

Unable to breath or sleep, he was going through oxygen at an enormous rate. Inhaling it constantly, he used up to four tanks a day. Soon, he couldn't walk even a few steps or get out of a chair without assistance. He was no longer able to cook for himself or even go to the bathroom unescorted.

Meanwhile a frantic effort was underway to get the Strodival before it was too late. Rilling's shipment had been sent parcel post and it appeared it would arrive posthumously if at all. My father's ex-wife Paula located the manufacturer of the drug and his chelation doctor kindly wrote the prescription.

Stalled by the language barrier, I found a German woman who could call Herbert Pharmaceuticals in Weisbaden to place the order to be shipped Federal Express. While I got busy in California, Paula was working on the problem from Minneapolis. She hired a translator in New York and had her own order sent out via Airborne Express.

We each tracked our precious packages through the ins-and-outs of international shipping while my father anxiously waited, fearing each hour would be his last.

The night before the Strodival was promised to arrive, my father wrote, "Will it come tomorrow? Is my time running out? My systems are failing..."

Sleep was just a memory. There was no reprieve from the constant struggle for breath, the insidious discomfort and the din of his own concern. This waking nightmare wore down his indomitable spirit. My father, the eternal optimist, was starting to crumble under the strain.

The morning my package was due to arrive, I was notified it had been seized by the FDA in Memphis for a routine inspection. Since we had the proper documentation they expected it to pass. But, by delaying this emergency medical shipment, I feared the FDA had just signed my father's death warrant.

Working the phones, Paula found her package was being routed through customs in New York where she had strings she could pull.

Paula's brother-in-law owned an import-export company. He was able to intercept the package and walk it through customs. He made it just in time to put the package on the last flight to Orange County.

With the Strodival safely on its way, we still couldn't breath a sigh of relief because Dad wasn't sure he could wait. Nothing frightened me more than watching him give up. It was like trying to keep someone from falling asleep in the freezing cold.

A KISS FOR THE DYING

Watching Paula pleading with him to hold on a little longer, my mind wandered back to when I first learned fathers are mortal.

My grandfather died without a goodnight kiss. To my dad, who was only 9 years old, that was the most horrible way to die. He'd had a fight with Grandfather the night before he died and, out of childish anger, lost his last chance to show his father how much he loved him. The boy felt responsible – as if that kiss could have shielded his father from the brain hemorrhage that took his life.

Between quarterbacking football games and dancing with pretty girls like my mother, my father spent much of his youth in the basement reading the books his father had collected before he died. He went on to become a writer himself. In later years, he realized that rather than exploring great literature, he'd been down there looking for his father.

To keep us from ever having the same regrets, Dad made sure each of his five children kissed him goodnight no matter what was happening, how we felt or how old we got. I never forgot the story of his father's death or the sadness with which he told it. I could almost see the snowflakes swirling drunkenly to the ground outside the window as the little boy stood alone by his father's coffin in the dark parlor.

My youngest brother, Colin, was only 9 years old when Dad had his heart attack. It was the summer of 1978. He underwent an emergency coronary double bypass operation. Determined that history not repeat itself, he made it through the surgery with flying colors.

Not long after he was discharged from the hospital, the replaced artery clogged. His strength drained away while the doctors assured us he was doing just fine. We watched helplessly as our vibrant, gregarious father became an old man at 42. He, who used to play tackle football with the kids and our St. Bernard, was now too fragile to touch.

Until those dark days, ours had been a happy house to grow up in. A hopeless romantic, my father would grab my mother when she was cooking dinner, whirl her around the kitchen table and dip her near the stove – all the while crooning some off-key tune in her ear. Each night I fell asleep to the sound of my mother laughing at my father's jokes.

While we were growing up, Dad worked as a freelance writer. I read an article once that said out of several thousand freelancers in the U.S., only a handful made a living. Dad raised five children on a rambling Wisconsin farm with a little Irish luck and a lot of macaroni and cheese dinners.

With rolling hills and thick forests full of wild berries, the farm was a source of inspiration but not income. Dad was a writer who dabbled in farming but harvested little more than peace and quiet. Nothing ever grew in his garden except weeds and the livestock was anything but domesticated.

The horse was too wild to be ridden and the dog ran away with the goat. Determined to find an animal he could domesticate, Dad took all the kids to a cattle auction. Caught up in the excitement, we lost our heads and bid on a milk cow. When Mom found out, she made us take it back.

Dad brought enthusiasm and humor to everything he did whether it be bottle-feeding calves, concocting his famous spaghetti sauce or writing up a new ad campaign. He laughed loud and he played hard. He was charming, fun and heartbreakingly sincere.

Snow came in October the year Dad's bypass failed. It blanketed the landscape and seemed to smother his energy. He'd get up late in the morning and try to stay awake until nap time.

The doctors had nothing to offer but another bypass. The first one hadn't worked and he had neither the strength nor the stomach for another. In desperation, he turned to a folk remedy recommended by a friend – Cayenne red pepper.

Cayenne saved my Dad's life. It cleared his clogged arteries, boosted circulation and restored his strength. As he was fond of saying, it put lead in his pencil. It brought him back to life and he felt better than ever before. He exuded vitality. With Cayenne as his constant companion, he put 1,000 miles on his bike every summer and had more energy than men half his age.

Left for dead by his doctor, he defied the odds. Every so often, we'd get a letter from the hospital informing him that one of his classmates in the physical therapy program had passed away and inquiring if he was dead yet. He always wrote back, telling him about the wonders of Cayenne, but they never responded.

Thanks to Cayenne and other heart healing herbs, my father lived to see his 9-year-old son Colin grow up, graduate from college and get married. He got to know his grandchildren; traveled to Europe and wrote a book about his experiences that he knew would make his father proud.

Ironically, the release of his book titled *Left for Dead* kicked off a chain of events that culminated in the doctor's diagnosis of end-stage heart failure. His wonderfully enthusiastic headlong plunge into publishing wore him out as he tried to take care of everybody but himself.

Like the Johnny Appleseed of Cayenne pepper, he set out to spread the word about herbal alternatives to heart surgery. With his natural charm and genuine concern for people, he became an instant celebrity – a health starlet of sorts.

He was on-call round the clock. The phone rang constantly. Radio interviews started at dawn and people with health problems called long after midnight. In the fall of '93, he hit the road. Promoting himself like a one-man rock band, he went on grueling cross-country book tours lasting several months at a time without a single roadie to carry his books.

Since the book was more of a mission than a money-making venture, he'd drive 400 miles just to talk to 10 people if he felt he could make a difference. He pushed on from Altoona to San Antonio, carting heavy boxes of books, grabbing meals at fast-food joints and collapsing on a different motel bed every night.

He gave of himself until there was nothing left. Finally, his heart faltered and his workaholic ways crashed in on him.

Cayenne had kept him going long after others would have dropped from exhaustion. But there came a time when the pungent red powder could no longer make up for a poor diet, lack of sleep, little exercise and a high stress lifestyle.

Cayenne had given my father a second chance at life back in 1978 when his bypass failed. Like the hero in an old Western, he rode off into the sunset with his trusty peppers by his side. What he didn't know is that just beyond the horizon congestive heart failure waits in ambush for people who've had heart attacks, clogged arteries or high blood pressure.

It takes more than Cayenne's "magic bullet" to get out alive. He could have headed congestive heart failure off at the pass with the help of a good diet, regular exercise, stress management, herbs and heart healthy supplements like calcium, magnesium, vitamins E and C, Coenzyme Q-10 and L-Carnitine.

Instead, my father walked blindly into heart failure and it was like falling into an open grave on a moonless night. The sides were too high to climb out.

Because of his aversion to doctors and his selfless attitude, he was in the final stages of heart failure before it was diagnosed and treatment could begin. Both sides of his heart were failing, water was filling his body from his ankles to his lungs and his heart was beating like a large winged bird caught in a tiny cage.

To top it all off, they later discovered he had an aortic aneurysm that was noted during his bypass operation but not revealed. It started out as a small bulge in the wall of the main artery.

From the age of 42 to 59 the time bomb in his chest grew bigger and bigger, distending and thinning the walls of his aorta. A hard mass formed in the center forcing the heart to work harder to push the blood through to the rest of the body. His blood pressure inched higher while the walls of his artery weakened. It was like blowing up a balloon to the breaking point.

Tests of his kidney function showed his blood pressure had been elevated for some time. If he'd had an occasional check-up with a doctor or herbalist or even used the drug store blood pressure machines, he might have caught it earlier and been able to lower his blood pressure with herbs, diet and stress reduction before it could trigger heart failure. Higher doses of Hawthorn could have restored the elasticity of his blood vessels to keep his blood pressure from going up. It also would have strengthened his circulatory system, helping to protect his heart from harm. "Hawthorn fixes broken hearts," Dad was fond of saying.

Herbs need time to work but we didn't find out the clock was ticking away Dad's life until the 11th hour. We bought time for herbs like Hawthorn to work with conventional treatment. For my father, a harsh critic of American drug-based medicine, taking heart medication was like selling his soul to the devil.

The day he was diagnosed with heart failure, Dec. 9, 1994, my father started taking a combination of prescription and herbal diuretics. Although he lost more than 6 pounds of water over that first weekend, it wasn't enough to get him out of danger. By Monday, he reluctantly agreed to go into the hospital for the first time in 16 years to "get drained."

To him, hospitals were where you go to die. Most of the people he knew who'd gone into the hospital, never made it out.

When you climb into a hospital bed, you don't automatically give up the right to make your own health care decisions. While his doctor respected his right to make informed, independent choices, we soon found out the on-call cardiologist had a bit of a "God complex."

The doctor had told us Dad's heart rate had split into two separate beats. The upper atrial rate drummed out at 300 beats per minute while the lower ventricle rate hovered around 130. Banging around in his chest in a lopsided frenzy, his heart was tearing itself apart.

When drugs failed to regulate his heart rhythm, the consulting cardiologist opted for a procedure called a cardioversion. Cardioversion uses electric shock to stop, then re-start the heartbeat in sync to the natural rhythm. The only problem is, sometimes it's easier to stop the heart than it is to re-start it.

Without explaining the dangers of the procedure, the

heart surgeon steamrolled my opinionated but exhausted father into allowing him to "jump start" his heart.

The "jump start" technique didn't sound like a good idea to me since the doctor had told us it was a miracle my father's overworked heart was still beating at all. I was concerned his heart couldn't take the shock.

His staff assured me the cardiologist would answer my concerns before he performed the procedure. When none of my calls were returned, I went to the hospital to track the cardiologist down. I arrived two hours before Dad's scheduled cardioversion.

As I walked through door, I bumped into the cardiologist who was congratulating himself on a job well done. Confirming my fear that my father could have died during the procedure – and he would have died alone – the cardiologist shrugged. "What does it matter now? It worked," he said and walked away as if he'd already dismissed the matter from his mind.

Happy to be alive, Dad was discharged from the hospital and going home at last.

Home was the sunny little Southern California beach town of San Clemente. Divorced from my mother, he'd left the harsh midwest winters behind once and for all when he realized his second marriage was also over.

Since then he'd "gone native," decking himself out in khaki shorts, multi-pocket shirts with epaulets, a straw hat with a tropical band and Birkenstock sandals paired with white athletic socks.

Every day until he got sick he'd put on his hat, slip on his sandals and hike up the hill to town where he'd pick out a fresh carnation for his lapel before crossing the street to the Calypso coffee shop to drink iced cappuccino, eat tuna salad and devour the *New York Times*.

Now that he'd made it out of the hospital, he was anxious to get back to his routine. His health was still shaky but he had his arsenal of herbs, supplementary medications, an exercise regime and his precious independence. There was no keeping him down.

A couple days after he got home, I went to visit him and found him gone. I couldn't believe it. He was supposed to be convalescing, waiting for visitors like me, not off gallivant-ing around. Here was someone who obviously didn't know how to be sick!

I knew he was too weak to get far on foot so I called Ginny the cab driver to track down my wayward Dad. I found him sipping iced tea at the Tropicana Bar and Grill. Watching him chat with the gang, you'd never know how close he'd come to dying just a few days ago.

It wasn't long before he was back to his old workaholic ways. Tired and breathless, he'd summon the energy to do a 6 a.m. radio show or listen patiently to a litany of someone else's health problems.

More often than not, Ginny the cab driver brought him down to the bar to watch Notre Dame games or catch a quick shark taco.

Concentrating on his recovery, he had concocted herbal formulas to fix himself. For "Dick's Heart Formula," he mixed 60 percent of hard-to-get Lily of the Valley with 20 percent Hawthorn, 15 percent Rosemary and 5 percent Cayenne. He supplemented it with Valerian, Kelp, Mother-wort, Ginger, Garlic, Bilberry and extra doses of Hawthorn extract.

Aside from herbs, he was building heart strength with vitamins, minerals, amino acids and hormones. Basically, if we heard it might work, he was taking it.

With the herbs and the medications, more sleep and healthier eating habits, he was slowly getting better. He started work on a new book to warn over 200,000 readers of *Left For Dead* about congestive heart failure and hope-fully, keep them from falling into the same painful trap. He was fighting his way out and by sharing his experience, he hoped to help others – just as he did in *Left For Dead*.

Tapping away on his word processor, he let the book take hold of his mind and a new sense of purpose lifted his spirits. Buoyed by high hopes, his condition improved day by day.

By the end of January, six weeks after his diagnosis, he felt good enough to gamble. It was then that he made the decision to stop taking Digitalis. With that roll of the dice he lost all the progress he'd made and began a downward slide only the Strodival could check.

SAVED BY STRODIVAL

Together and separately, Paula and I tried to persuade my father to hang on until my sister got back from the airport with the Strodival. We joked to distract him, we challenged him to bring out his stubborn streak, we even prodded him into energy-giving anger and finally, we pleaded our selfish desire to keep him with us a little while longer.

The minutes crawled by with agonizing slowness. Finally, the Strodival arrived. He took one, waited 10 minutes and took another. Almost immediately, his breathing became more regular. His voice regained its timbre and hope lit up his eyes once again.

With the crisis past, we laughed when my shipment finally arrived the next morning. But I know if it hadn't been for Paula and her connections, we would have been mourning my father's death that day instead.

"The Strodival crisis," as we called it, revealed that sheer willpower was keeping my father alive. He'd put all his faith in that German medicine and it was almost as if he willed it to work.

All natural systems of medicine revolve around the belief that health is a manifestation of your physical, mental and emotional state. You can strengthen the body, but you won't be truly well unless you can also nurture the mind and soothe the soul. So much of feeling good comes from attitude and outlook.

Hope is the best medicine. A positive attitude is the purest therapy. You can't bottle it, box it or patent it but by understanding it, you can promote it, build it and encourage it.

Everyone, whether they are young or old, healthy or ill, needs to feel useful, attractive and special. Sick people probably need that kind of self-esteem even more. To help my father meet these needs, we concentrated on the parts we played in the drama that was his life.

His ex-wife Paula had always swooned over his charm and marveled at his quick wit. She catered to his every need, making him feel handsome, interesting and admired.

Al, his friend of 13 years, brought out the man he was – a daring risk-taker who still had more adventures ahead of him. They had worked together, traveled together, argued politics together and laughed together. Al reminded him of all the things he'd done and left him looking forward to the things they'd do once he was well again.

As for me, I respected him enough to let him make his own decisions. I found it's very tempting to treat a sick parent like a child. It's demeaning to an adult and may be one reason why many people don't last long in nursing homes. The best way to take care of a parent is to let them think they're still capable of taking care of you. (But thank goodness they don't have to anymore!)

I always insisted on being allowed to live my own life and make my own decisions – good and bad. Now, I had to show my father the same respect no matter how frightened I was by the course he was likely to take. For example, I knew if the time came, I'd have to honor his request not to be resuscitated.

For his part, my father had a few revelations during the "Strodival Crisis." His journal entry reflected not only his determination to regain his health on his own terms but his understanding of the toll it might take on others. "Get used to kindness," he wrote. "You owe it to help others. This is not the will of God. Fight to the end."

We got ready for a long hard fight. In the words of Dylan Thomas, "Do not go gentle into that good night."

Despite regular doses of Strodival and Digitalis, Dad was so weak by late February he needed oxygen round-the-clock. Sluggish circulation began to affect his body and his mind. He had trouble moving around, digesting his food and keeping his thoughts straight.

He started to experience sporadic short-term memory loss when not enough blood made it to his brain. He had trouble remembering to eat and to take his medication. He couldn't stand up long enough to cook and he couldn't recall if he'd left the stove on.

My father was sharp enough to know when his thinking wasn't right. He chronicled some of his worst moments of confusion in his journal: "Inventing words, tunes, yet couldn't talk. No fever but hallucinations. Thought (the apartment had) a back porch, upstairs, an extra bedroom and a room next to the kitchen."

Based on blood flow, Dad's disorientation could come

and go at any time of the day or night. Treasuring his privacy, he didn't like the idea of having people watching over him all the time but it was obvious he needed someone to cook his meals and monitor his medication. After all, we'd already found out that too little Digitalis can be just as deadly as too much.

Since I had a full-time job and Paula and Al were only able to visit, I decided to hire a nurse. The local service sent over their best and brightest. Expecting an efficient grandmother-type in crisp whites, I was in for a pleasant surprise.

MINISTRATIONS OF NURSES AND NUNS

The nurse's name was Steve. In his spare time, he was a body builder. The rest of the time, he was just a dream come true.

Tall, blonde and handsome, Steve was a competent nurse and a good companion. As a fitness buff, he shared my father's interest in natural remedies. Steve monitored his medication, took his blood pressure, cooked his meals, did the laundry, cleaned the house and listened with rapt attention to his experiences with herbs.

Steve was honest, conscientious and kind. Dad liked him immensely and looked forward to his daily visits. Knowing he was there put my mind at ease. In a journal, he logged the events of the day while I jotted down notes from each night. Together, we kept track of Dad's diet, medication, herbs and supplements, activities and attitude – trying to learn what worked and what didn't.

Medication proved to be both a blessing and a curse. Regular doses of Digitalis and Strodival helped keep my father alive, but the other drugs nearly killed him. They shook his heart rhythm, boosted his blood pressure and stole his sleep.

If there was a side-effect to be had, my father got it. The blood pressure medications raised his blood pressure dangerously high before dropping it again. The anti-arrhythmic drugs caused other rhythm disturbances to develop so that after awhile, Dad's heart had played every beat from hard rock to reggae.

The chemical diuretics worked best at night – robbing him of precious sleep. The prescription sedatives wouldn't wear off by the time he needed to wake up.

He was put on Procardia, a Calcium Channel Blocker that federal health officials warn is responsible for twice as many deaths as other drugs in its class, and Quinidine, an anti-arrhythmic drug that studies show is more likely to kill you than if you took nothing at all. Vasotec, an ACE Inhibitor, had to be used in just the right amount or it caused a violent barking cough that threatened to rupture his aortic aneurysm. We stuck mainly to Digitalis and Strodival.

Over the course of his illness, my father had half a dozen doctors with specialties ranging from cardiology to chelation. They all meant well but they made some rather deadly mistakes.

With the best of intentions, his first doctor gave him a drug we later discovered could cause lupus, an autoimmune disease where the body attacks itself, destroying healthy tissue. Another doctor switched him to an easy-to-take liquid form of Lanoxin (Digitalis) but accidentally prescribed the children's dose. Underdosing on Digitalis would have killed him by inches.

It seemed like you had to be a chemist to figure out the right mix or a mad scientist concocting formulas in the stomach rather than a test tube. Drug interactions were discovered purely by accident. The doctors either neglected to warn us or they just didn't know – even though it's in the Physician's Desk Reference (PDR).

For example, mindful of his high blood pressure and cholesterol levels, Steve and I shifted Dad from his favorite breakfast of bacon and eggs to oatmeal and fruit. Months later, we learned that oat bran interferes with the absorption of Digitalis – his most critical drug.

None of his doctors said anything about oatmeal or the fact that over-the-counter antacids – which he ate like candy – also interact with Lanoxin. The ibuprofen he took for his aching back negates the effects of ACE Inhibitors like the Vasotec he was taking.

More trusted than his medication were the kinder, gentler

heart herbs and supplements that made up the bulk of his treatment. He was on daily doses of L-Carnitine, melatonin, Co-Enzyme Q-10, magnesium, zinc, silica, thiamin and vitamins C, E, beta carotene and a B complex formula that included B1, B2, B6, B12, niacin, biotin, pantothenic acid and folic acid. One of his doctors also had him on a hormone therapy consisting of DHEA and knife-tip doses of powdered testosterone.

To complete his repertoire, he took the herbal heart tonic he concocted with Lily of the Valley, Hawthorn, Rosemary and Cayenne. He added supplemental doses of Hawthorn, Valerian, Motherwort, Garlic, Ginger and Kelp. If he looked like he was retaining water again, we'd drop in herbal diuretics including Dandelion leaf and root, Burdock root and Cornsilk.

At its peak, his regimen contained 94 different pills. Over time, it would wreak havoc with his digestive system. Wherever possible, we shifted from capsules and tablets to liquid forms of the herbs and supplements. We changed his diet – as much as he would let us – to make it more nutritious, easily digestible and less acidic.

Al was the only one who ever had any lasting influence over Dad's eating habits. He made trying new supplements and healthier foods fun.

When Dad got sick, Al flew out to California to help him ring in the New Year and left him in the habit of juicing. Juicing vegetables and fruits enabled my father to get more nutrition with less strain on his sluggish digestive system.

Picking up Al's lead, my brother Devin came out for a visit and concocted his own brand of "killer juice." Made from fresh beets, carrots, melon, ginger and three cloves of garlic, one sip knocked you right out of your shoes! Dad loved it.

While Devin was a genius with juice, Barbara was a macrobiotic miracle worker. Barbara, who became Dad's nurse after Steve moved with his wife to Texas, was into cooking, chanting and channeling. She helped design Dad's new macrobiotic menu.

After introducing juice to Dad's diet, Al had discovered that macrobiotic foods like Miso soup, twig tea, green tea and Japanese Ume plum could make the blood more alkaline.

The prevailing European medical theory blames heart disease on thick acidic blood. Acidic blood is caused by toxins in medication and diets high in sugar, simple carbohydrates, animal protein and citrus fruits. For those with congestive heart failure, highly acidic blood can cause crushing fatigue and damage healthy heart tissue.

With Barbara in the kitchen, breakfast might be Buckwheat pancakes flavored with Umi plum. Lunch was warm and soothing Miso soup with bits of carrot and scallion. Dinner could feature garlic-seared calamari with a Tamari-Shoyu sauce.

It was quite a departure for my father who referred to himself half-jokingly as "Mr. Cheeseburger" and boasted of being "a nutritionist's nightmare." During one radio interview, Dad explained his long-held views on nutrition.

"Some of my best friends are vegetarians, but it doesn't work for me. I eat what I want," he said. "When my body sends the meat signal, I eat it. Sometimes it sends for eggs, fish, spaghetti, turkey (dark meat, please), fried chicken (with the skin on), baked potatoes – my body likes nearly everything. It usually wants tuna salad for lunch."

Like most people, his eating habits reflected his upbringing – but it didn't mean he wasn't willing to try new things. When I was a kid, we boycotted tuna to save the dolphins, passed up cold cuts and hot dogs because sodium nitrate was linked to cancer and ate ice cream for breakfast.

The ice cream phase, which was one of my favorites, came about after Dad read an article on the poor nutritional content of breakfast cereal. In the study, one group of rats ate the cereal, while another group ate the box it came in. The rats that ate the box turned out to be healthier than their fellow cereal-eating vermin. After that, breakfast was sundaes, shakes and cones rather than krispies, flakes or pops. He figured at least then we'd be getting our daily dairy requirement.

As part of his enjoyment of life, Dad ate with gusto. He loved to cook everything from rich beef stroganoff to crispy fried chicken. When times were good, we celebrated with bags of tiny square fast-food hamburgers called White Castles and handfuls of greasy onion rings.

Dad's diet couldn't have been worse but it's hard to know better. Even the top nutritionists disagree as to what is really "heart smart." Now his condition was so delicate that indulging in chocolate cake or pudding and ice cream could cost him dearly. Sugary, rich or oily food caused severe indigestion, bloating and diarrhea. What started as a treat could now trigger days of misery.

I had never heard about this macrobiotic diet before Al introduced us to it, but I could see that it was really working for Dad.

Partially pre-digested, the fermented soybean paste that makes Miso soup was so easily absorbed, he had no problem with the indigestion and bloating that plagued him for months. The anti-oxidant action of the twig and green tea was revitalizing while the Ume Plum concentrate seemed to build back his strength.

Dispensed using a tiny one gram spoon, the 1.4 ounce jar of Umi plum concentrate actually contains a whole kilo of fresh plums. It had been used for centuries in Japan to invigorate emperors, warriors and athletes. It seemed to be doing the same job for Dad so we put it in everything we could.

While his diet was coming together he got a craving for a little food for the soul. An Irish Catholic, Dad wasn't what you'd call a regular church-goer. We'd usually oversleep, arrive late and have to stand in the back. Still, he was a former alter boy, although he said, "They'd take anyone in those days!"

My sister put in a call to Our Lady of Fatima – the Irish Catholic church with the Spanish name. They sent Sister Theresa Kelly and after an hour of talking to her under the San Clemente sun, my father proclaimed her the most charming woman he had ever met.

The feeling was mutual. A native of the Emerald Isle, Sister Theresa Kelly had a lilting Irish brogue and a soothing manner. Dad eagerly anticipated her visits, often donning a fresh carnation for the occasion.

Unfortunately, the delightful Irish nun wasn't always able to come in person. Caught up in her duties at the convent, she hand-picked parishioners to drop in on my father. After awhile, I noticed that one man in particular was sent.

At the memorial, I heard Sister Theresa Kelly whispering the reason to Dad's ex-wife Paula.

"I had to start sending a man because he was charming all the ladies," she said hiding a smile behind her hand.

No matter how he was feeling, my father always greeted ladies with a compliment and men with a handshake. He even had a kind word for the paramedics when they arrived.

GREETINGS AND GOOD NEWS

Since the quality of Dad's life had improved with the new diet and his treatment regimen, I was stunned when I came to his apartment one hot July afternoon and found him curled up on the floor, gasping for breath.

While he was reading the paper, joking with friends on the phone and monitoring the O.J. trial from his armchair, his chest had been filling with fluid. Hidden behind his rib cage, the crushing weight of the water eventually collapsed his lung.

As the trustee of his Living Will, I knew of his strong aversion to hospitals, doctors and drugs so I actually asked him if he minded if I called an ambulance now. I had called my doctor, the one who'd diagnosed Dad's heart failure, and he told me that if I tried to take him in my car, he could go into cardiac fatigue – which would be the same as cardiac arrest.

Dad kindly agreed to be taken to the hospital by ambulance. I asked them to come in without lights and sirens so as not to alarm him. Coming in quietly as promised, the two burly paramedics hoisted him onto a stretcher. As they were strapping him in I heard them ask how he was feeling.

So weak he could barely open his eyes, he smiled and said casually, "Well, I've been better. How are you?"

In the emergency room, my doctor tried to prepare me for the possibility that Dad might not live through the night. I'd heard that one before. And I knew somehow I would hear it again. Soon, I wouldn't be able to count the number of times on one hand.

What they didn't know, was that my Dad had nicknamed himself "the original Come-back Kid." He would never say die, he always fought his way back. He delighted in doing what people said couldn't be done.

Doctors drained the fluid from his chest cavity by inserting a catheter through his back and sucking it out. It was a painful process but nothing compared to the agony of coughing the sticky red fluid out of the collapsed right lung. I guess that's where the phase "coughing your lungs out" comes from.

By the time he was brought to his room, he was trembling with fatigue. With tubes in his arms and nose, he still insisted on shaking hands with his male nurse and making the proper introductions. In his life, he never compromised on ethics, principles or etiquette. I sat with him until he fell asleep.

In the morning, not only was he still alive, he was impatiently waving people out of the way of the TV – he was watching the O.J. trial. Al, who traveled all night to be by his side, had to wait until the commercial break to hear his side of the story.

We sat around chatting as if we were back in Dad's living room listening to Paula puttering in the kitchen rather than the beep of a heart monitor. After awhile, the doctor came by and we stepped outside to let him examine Dad. When he came out, he motioned us to follow him down the hall.

In a halting voice, the doctor told us that X-rays revealed Dad had an aortic aneurysm that had grown to 7 centimeters – about the size of a tangerine. Anything over 5 centimeters calls for emergency surgery, the doctor said, because it could rupture at any time. Like a time bomb in his chest, if the aneurysm exploded, he'd have only seconds to live.

Staggered by the news, Al and I went back in to see how my father was taking it. Looking up from his stack of newspapers, Dad smiled brightly. "Did you hear?" he said. "Great news!"

My jaw must have dropped to my knees. I couldn't for the life of me figure out how he could find anything to celebrate about what seemed to me to be a death sentence. I asked him to enlighten me.

He said his greatest fear was becoming a burden, a vegetable – "poor uncle Dick in the back room." Heart failure had proven to be more tenacious than heart disease. It was harder to shake off than a pit bull. Just when you thought you had it licked, it'd "come back around and bite you in the ass," he said.

Sometimes it seemed for each step forward, he took two steps back. He figured with the aneurysm, death would be mercifully quick – like stepping in front of a speeding train. Then, he wouldn't face the despair of being trapped in a body he could no longer control.

Although the doctor said it might be possible to operate on the aneurysm if it wasn't too close to the heart, Dad was against heart surgery of any kind. His reason could have been the failed bypass that re-shaped his life or he may have known he was so frail by the time the aneurysm was discovered the chances were high he would die on the table. Whatever his reasons, his mind was made up.

To get the energy to make it out of the hospital, Dad's body metabolized all his fat and most of his muscle. He went home all skin and bones.

Sitting on the couch sipping beer with Al with his hat askew and his clothes hanging on him, he looked like a talking scarecrow. Watching him, I felt fear and admiration. He got himself home through sheer determination and you could see just by looking how much it had cost him.

My doctor gracefully bowed out of Dad's case after he refused the surgery to correct the aneurysm. He said he thought we needed to find a doctor closer to home in case of a likely emergency. I had already hired a nurse who lived around the corner to take over 24-hour care of my increasingly frail father.

Mariann reminded me of a feisty, no-nonsense grandmother dressed up in baggy overalls and giant hoop earrings. A nurse for 30 years, she'd seen it all and nothing fazed her. She was just as opinionated as my Dad. She always had something to say – whether he wanted to hear it or not. She drove him to distraction, and her choice of vehicle was a bright orange VW bug.

He improved greatly under her careful watch. It was hard to tell if he got better so he could be rid of her or if she was just the right medicine. Although he often accused her of treating him like a child – and he was justified – she never babied him.

The problem was, his illness was like a crazy roller coaster ride. He could be incapacitated and incoherent one day and wake up clear-headed and energetic the next. When he was desperately sick, he was grateful for her all-encompassing efficiency but when he was well, he re-asserted his independence. So they went along, clashing and complementing each other.

For her part, Mariann watched over him and protected him from outside stress. She admired him greatly and virtually adopted the rest of the family. She was honest, reliable and ready for anything.

To give both of them a break, I came up as often as I could. Mariann had weeks off when Al or Paula came to visit. In the meantime, to fill in the gaps and keep Dad from getting bored or lonely, I tapped into his vast store of friends. He was the kind of guy who needed projects and people in the same way the rest of us need food and water to survive.

FRIENDS IN FAR AWAY PLACES

His friend Cory once said my father collected characters like refrigerator magnets. He attracted all kinds – nuns and gigolos, mercenaries and merchants, celebrities and poets. He'd listen with the same earnest interest to a child's chatter as he would to an adult conversation.

You could drop my father into a crowded cocktail party or a jungle gathering and he would find something in common to talk about. I knew that for a fact. I still have the postcard he sent me from Peru when he was down there talking to a band of cut-throat mercenaries.

In between writing jobs, Dad started the monkey business. When the opportunity came his way, Mom was 7 months pregnant with my brother Foley, my sister Kelly and I were toddling age and brother Devin was a dream for the future. Without hesitation, she told him to go ahead with his plan to sell squirrel monkeys through the mail.

Dad flew down to the Amazon to work a deal with the mercenaries for them to gather monkeys when the rainy season put a temporary end to war. Back then, commercial flights into Lima were virtually unknown. He took cargo planes and puddle jumpers that still had the camouflage paint from their army days.

Using his college Spanish and a lot of charisma, he managed to speak the mercenaries' language. He forged a deal with the force of his personality that held until he left the business a couple of years later.

Black with furry white beards, the tiny squirrel monkeys looked like charming little old men. In reality, they were wild and vicious. Dad decided to get out after he had to call animal control to remove one from the home of a 65-year-old woman in Iowa. Business was booming, but that didn't matter to Dad if there was even a remote possibility someone might be hurt or disappointed.

A few months after Dad went back to writing, one of his mercenary friends left him a token of their esteem. The thought was there, but some gifts from the wilds of the Amazon don't go over well in the farmlands of Wisconsin.

Every morning, Kelly and I would go out and play in the front yard while our mother made breakfast. That day, for some reason, Mom went out with us. If she hadn't, I might not have been around to write about it. Relaxing in the sun was a fully grown python with a red bow around its neck.

Being curious, I'm sure we would have investigated the flash of red and we'd have been breakfast for that snake in the grass. Pythons that size have been known to swallow cattle whole and, at age 3 and 4, we were basically bite-size.

When my mom calmed down, she called the Como Park Zoo in St. Paul and had Dad's new pet carted away. I don't think he ever missed it. It was just another sign of his popularity among people of all ages, occupations and backgrounds.

Dad accepted people for who they were and respected their dreams. He made them feel good about themselves and want to be everything he saw in them. He might have spent his life looking for his father but, in doing so, he found the best in everyone around him.

FIELD TRIPS AND FIREWORKS

Still a gregarious host, most of the time he was so weak, people had to come to him. Charlie, his friend and former business partner, helped put on patio barbecues with a super secret sauce that required three days to make. His nieces, nephew and neighbors dropped in for a snack and a chat. The phone rang with calls from friends near and far.

When he was feeling better, Paula, Al or I would take him on "field trips." We'd put the top down on the convertible and drive up the coast, sip a beer on the pier or head over to the coffee shop for cappuccino and conversation with the locals. He'd made a lot of friends in San Clemente and when he was able to get out, they flocked to him.

Despite constant discomfort and daily frustration, his smile was always ready and his outlook was optimistic. "You've got to plan for life," he explained. "Death will take care of itself."

Time and time again, he rose above his illness. He had heart failure – it didn't have him.

For weeks before he was rushed to the hospital with a collapsed lung, we had been planning to watch the Fourth of July fireworks from the pier. But when we arrived to take him there, he was too sick to make the short trip.

Disheartened, he decided to stay inside and watch television. I knew he'd regret letting heart failure ruin his Fourth of July festivities and I also knew this might be the last time he enjoyed the bright beauty of fireworks against the night sky.

So, my friend Scott and I set up a private viewing in the driveway complete with his easy chair, blankets and oxygen. Weighing little more than I did by this time, he was too wobbly on his feet to make it down the stairs so Scott half-carried him. Dropping exhausted into his chair, he was soon beaming – exhilarated by the light show.

CHOOSING BETWEEN LIFE AND DEATH

A month after the fireworks faded, the water came back. Once again, Dad's chest cavity had filled with fluid. He was drowning in it.

Only a week before, on July 24, he'd felt so much better,

he'd written a note to himself in the shaky scrawl that had become his handwriting, "Letter to all radio stations: I'm back!"

Now he was so weak he couldn't eat or even get out of bed. I could see the water sloshing from one side of his chest to the other. I called my doctor – the one who'd cared for him the last time. He advised me to get Dad a new doctor by taking him to the nearest hospital. He also told me it was time to let my father choose whether he wanted to live under these conditions or die.

At first I was shocked that he would suggest giving up as an option. But then I remembered my father always told me (and anyone who would listen), "I'm doing the dying."

I hated hearing him say it, but what he meant was that he wanted be just as much in control of how he died as he'd always been of how he lived. His body was betraying him now, but his mind was always his own. To take that away would have killed his spirit. I had made a promise to always tell him the truth and let him make his own decisions and I had to honor it.

I went back into his dimly lit bedroom and sat on the edge of his bed. He listened quietly as I laid it all out. His brown eyes never left my face as I explained that he would die if he didn't go the hospital now, but that wouldn't fix the problem. Without a heart transplant, the water would just keep coming back and he'd have to go the hospital every two or three weeks to be drained.

I asked him again if he wanted to get in line for a heart transplant. His answer – as always – was no. Speaking slow to keep my voice from shaking, I told him he needed to decide if he wanted to let the doctors save his life now and sign up for regular "draining sessions" to keep him going as long as we could. I don't think I exhaled until he said yes.

I don't know if you should ever offer anyone the option to die but at least he was the one to make the choice to live.

He wasn't himself in the hospital. Disoriented by the drugs, poor cerebral circulation and strange surroundings, he told my friend Jennifer and everyone who called or came to visit that he'd hurt himself working round-the-clock shifts in an underwear factory. It was a colorful fabrication, full of detail – and absolutely unshakable. He would listen to my explanation of what really happened and then turn calmly to the person next to me and launch into his tale.

He came out of his mental malaise a couple of days before he was to leave the hospital. His release was delayed when doctors thought his aneurysm might be leaking. He was prepared for emergency surgery, but he refused to go under the knife.

His new doctor admitted that in his current condition, Dad had less than a 40 percent chance of surviving the surgery and he would still wake up to heart failure. Under the circumstances, the doctor admitted he probably wouldn't do it either, but said that without the surgery to fix the aneurysm, we'd never be able to beat the heart failure.

THEN CAME THE GENTLE NIGHT

We arrived home with a "drainage" schedule for Dad that would start in September. As for now, he seemed revitalized by his hospital stay. He and Mariann had even come to a new understanding – a big improvement from the usual uneasy truce.

He began to appreciate her sense of humor and her loyalty. For her part, Mariann thought he was "the perfect patient." She admired his positive attitude and his uncompromising kindness.

"He's got his own ideas, but that's what you want because he's always trying – he never gives up," she told me. "He's the kind of man you want to do for."

Mariann volunteered to take him to his next doctor's appointment the Friday before Labor Day. He laughed when he told me about what a crazy driver she was, careening through Orange County traffic in her dented little VW Bug.

When I came to visit that night they looked happy together – like a couple of old friends rather than nurse and patient. Dad was in high spirits. He'd felt better in the past week than he had since January – before he dropped the Digitalis. He even let me beat him at a couple of games of Crazy 8s.

We'd been talking about new adventures to fill the three weeks between his drainage sessions. We knew from experience he'd have at least two weeks of good health, so that night we started planning a cruise for October. He wanted to go to Ireland – but there weren't any cruises there until spring so he settled for the warm waters of the Mediterranean.

We got out the brochures Paula had picked up for him and narrowed it down to two trips – the adventure cruise or the La Dulce Vita tour. It was either whisk Paula away for a shipboard romance or explore the Greek islands with Al. He was at a real crossroads but, like everything, it was his decision to make. My only advice was not to mix them up and take Al on the La Dulce Vita tour!

Leaving him dreaming about the possibilities, I went home for the weekend. Charlie was planning to throw Dad a Labor Day barbecue and Dad said he was looking forward to having some time to himself that Saturday and Sunday.

Sunday afternoon Mariann called. Dad had felt so good the night before he decided to do some sit-ups. Not a good idea for a guy with a huge aortic aneurysm. Now his groin area was hurting and he was afraid it was his hernia. He was also feeling sick to his stomach and he hadn't eaten anything all day.

I was relieved to hear the pain was in his groin because I knew back pain could mean the aneurysm was leaking. Little did I know groin pain and nausea were also symptoms of internal bleeding.

I asked Mariann to go get the ingredients and make him up a batch of Miso soup which had always soothed his stomach. I avoided the temptation to chide my father for those crazy sit-ups. Instead, I advised him to relax and rest up for Charlie's Labor Day visit.

I promised to call back later and come over if he needed me, otherwise I'd see about maybe crashing Charlie's barbecue. We would also call the doctor first thing Tuesday to see if we could have his hernia checked. He seemed happy with that and told me he was going to go take a nap. I told him I loved him but over the phone there could be no kiss goodnight.

I was just coming back from the beach when Mariann called to tell me my father had died.

She had gone to the store as I asked when it happened. His aneurysm ruptured and he died within seconds. Alone and without a goodnight kiss.

PART THREE

Standing by the baggage carousel in Minneapolis, I waited for my last suitcase to come into view. I was on my way to Dad's hometown of Faribault for his memorial service. In the bag on my shoulder, I had pictures to show from his days as a cab driver, a quarterback, a husband, a friend and a father.

Shifting around the crowd of passengers, I glanced at the gray-haired man next to me. He appeared to be in his late 60s. As my bag rounded the carousel, the man was joined by a younger woman. I could tell by the way he smiled at her she was his daughter.

Grabbing my bag, I turned away from the happy reunion wondering why some daughters are lucky enough to have their fathers live so long while others die too soon.

For those at risk, it takes more than luck to avoid heart failure. If we had realized back in 1978 how critical diet and lifestyle are to continuing heart health, my father might have avoided the trap of heart failure. Once in its grip, a survival guide like this one could have enhanced his quality of life and extended the time he had on earth. We can't change the past but we can use what we've learned to give others a future.

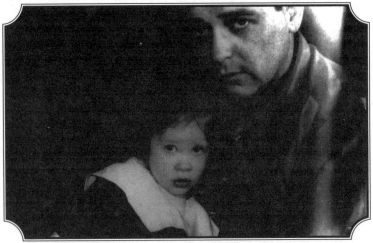

DICK HOLDS HIS DAUGHTER SHANNON, 2,
WHILE THEY WAIT THEIR TURN TO SEE SANTA CLAUS.

ANATOMY OF A KILLER

He who has health, has hope;
he who has hope, has everything.

-ARABIAN PROVERB

A GREAT LOSS

We had a funeral for my father, Dick Quinn, in his boyhood hometown of Faribault, Minnesota. It was beautiful, as funerals go. The sad thing about them is they make you realize how much you've just lost. This one was no exception.

The room was full of friends and family, all profoundly affected by his absence. A collage of pictures hinted at the magic that was Dick Quinn: a little boy in a cowboy outfit, a high school quarterback, husband, father and much more.

Among the family friends and relatives, I met a few people whose lives Dad had touched – with Cayenne.

"Your father saved my life," an elderly woman

proclaimed proudly. "I have congestive heart failure and I take Cayenne every day. I'm 83."

As she and her daughter ran to a garage sale conveniently located next door, a thought nagged at me.

"Why couldn't he save his own life?"

Here was a woman in her 80s, still very much alive, enjoying life and doing what she wanted – with congestive heart failure!

I know why.

Because he recovered from his heart attack and failed bypass operation, my father thought he had beaten heart disease. He didn't know about the condition that awaits the majority of heart attack survivors: Congestive Heart Failure (CHF).

We believe he had CHF for a couple years before he died. Looking back, we recognize the symptoms.

He explained these problems away: a bad cold, a hard bed, a pulled muscle from lugging books around an airport. It sounded very plausible. He was often on the run, undertaking grueling book tours lasting months at a time. Travel is, above all, tiring.

Even when he was home, he was always moving – meeting with someone and having radio interviews at dawn. He received phone calls at all hours from people needing advice for their health problems. He never had time to think about his own health. He didn't eat well. He didn't take time for himself – time to rest, exercise, time to just slow down.

It wasn't until he ended up in a hospital in December of '94 that he had to admit something was wrong. By the time he accepted that he had CHF and started to learn about it, it was very late. The tests showed his CHF had already progressed quite far – too far according to doctors who didn't even expect him to live through the night.

If he had listened to his body and taken care of himself, I know he would be here today. He would be alive and well and have many happy, productive years ahead of him.

That is the reason for this chapter. With early detection and the appropriate action, the progression of CHF can be halted and in many instances, reversed. But most of all, those who are at risk for CHF might be able to avoid the condition altogether.

THE RISE IN
CONGESTIVE HEART FAILURE

The number of people with congestive heart failure has risen dramatically in recent years. Over 400,000 new cases of CHF are diagnosed each year. It is estimated over 3 million Americans have CHF right now.

Congestive heart failure accounts for more hospital visits by people over the age of 65 than any other ailment. This year, over one million Americans will be hospitalized with CHF.

The huge increase in CHF cases is primarily because more and more people are surviving heart attacks. From 1950 to 1991, the death rate from heart attack has been cut in half. In just 10 years, from 1982 to 1992, the death rate from heart attack declined by 31.4 percent.

This good news is tempered by the likelihood of survivors developing CHF. Today's heart attack survivor may well be tomorrow's CHF patient. Within six years of a heart attack, 20 percent of patients will develop CHF. About 11.2 million people alive today have a history of heart attack or angina.

While huge strides have been made to increase the chance of survival for heart attack victims, the same can't be said for people with CHF. In fact, the problem is getting worse.

From 1979 to 1991, CHF mortality increased by 77.5 percent. Only half of the patients diagnosed with CHF live more than five years. Of those, only 15 percent of women survive longer than 8 to 12 years.

Life expectancy varies greatly and depends on many factors, including the degree of advancement of the condition, the underlying cause of the CHF and how effectively it is treated. These statistics are a call to action – a challenge to learn more about CHF and what can be done to reverse it or even avoid the condition altogether.

What is
Congestive Heart Failure

Congestive heart failure does not mean that your heart is "failing" or that it will stop completely. "Failure" means the heart is unable to meet the full demands of the body.

Simply put – the heart can't pump the amount of blood the body needs to function. The heart is running one step behind.

The inability of the heart to keep the blood moving properly causes congestion in the lungs and, later, in the other tissues of the body.

Blood cells are carried through the body in a liquid called plasma. One of the main ingredients of plasma is water. The pressure of the blood backing up from the damaged heart causes water to be forced out of the blood into the tissues.

The pooling of fluid in the tissues makes it harder for blood to circulate, raising blood pressure. This higher blood pressure, in turn, forces more water out of the blood and into the tissues. This vicious cycle accelerates the advancement of the condition.

How the Heart Works

About the size of your fist, the heart is a remarkable device. The average heart beats more than 85,000 times a day, circulating each blood cell through the body approximately 1,185 times.

To understand how it works, think of your heart as two separate two-stage pumps. One pump is the right atrium and right ventricle, and the other is the left atrium and left ventricle.

It is called "two-stage" because the two chambers work together. Blood enters the atrium which contracts, pumping it into the ventricle. This "tops off" the ventricle, assuring that it has a full charge of blood when it contracts, sending the blood on its way.

Even though these two pumps are separate, they work in unison. Both atriums and then both ventricles contract at

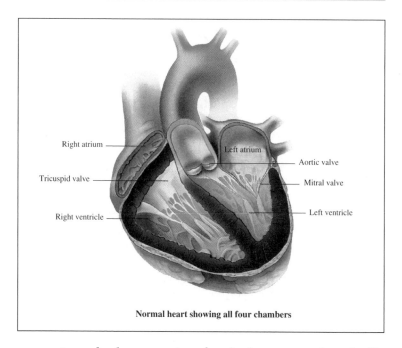

Normal heart showing all four chambers

Right atrium

Tricuspid valve

Right ventricle

Left atrium

Aortic valve

Mitral valve

Left ventricle

approximately the same time for the best strength and efficiency, circulating the blood from head to toe.

Returning from the body, the oxygen-depleted blood enters the right atrium, which contracts, sending it into the right ventricle. The right ventricle contracts, pushing the blood into the lungs, where it exchanges carbon dioxide for oxygen. The oxygen-rich blood then enters the left atrium, which contracts, pushing it into the left ventricle. Finally, the left ventricle contracts, sending the blood out through the aorta to arteries throughout the body.

Rhythm is vitally important to the proper functioning of the heart. The action of the ventricles and atriums are precisely coordinated to help each pump work in the most efficient and powerful way it can, providing your body with the blood it needs.

The heart is like a finely tuned sports car engine – all parts must work together in the correct sequence for the heart to function properly. While the heart can "run" with one or two chambers "misfiring," its performance is greatly diminished. It doesn't stop, but it just can't keep up.

THE IMPORTANCE OF A HEALTHY HEART

Each part of the human body, from your shinbone to your liver, is made up of cells. For your body to function properly, the cells must be healthy. An ample supply of oxygen- and nutrient-rich blood is essential.

Blood is the medium through which your cells receive the oxygen and nutrients they need. Just as important, blood also takes away the byproducts, namely wastes and toxins.

When the blood supply is not sufficient, the cells weaken. Toxins and wastes can build up, damaging the cells. Cell function is impaired and eventually, the cells can die.

A healthy heart pumps approximately 5-6 liters (one liter is about a quart) at rest, while a weakened heart pumps between 2½ and 3½ liters. Because pumping power is so critical, nature gives us all an early boost.

SYMPTOMS AND PROGRESSION OF HEART FAILURE

When we are born, nature gives our bodies a little extra capacity. Just like we have two kidneys when one can do the job, so are we born with extra pumping capacity in our hearts.

As we age, the heart can slowly lose some of its strength and efficiency. Those with healthy circulatory systems may never notice this decline. But, for those with congestive heart failure, as the heart's pumping power slowly decreases with age, its production begins to lag behind the needs of the body and the condition starts to materialize.

While there are many different causes of CHF, the progression of the condition follows one main course. CHF starts with the Asymptomatic stage, where the heart first begins to falter and the body attempts to compensate. This sets the stage for Left-sided failure, which is easily recognized by congestion in the lungs. The third and final stage is Right-sided failure, evidenced by the pooling of water in the ankles (edema).

CHF is a progressive condition. Each step along the way

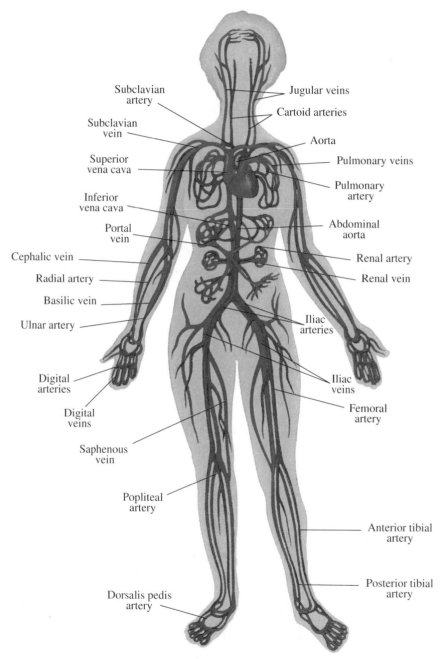

Subclavian artery
Subclavian vein
Superior vena cava
Inferior vena cava
Portal vein
Cephalic vein
Radial artery
Basilic vein
Ulnar artery
Digital arteries
Digital veins
Saphenous vein
Popliteal artery
Dorsalis pedis artery
Jugular veins
Cartoid arteries
Aorta
Pulmonary veins
Pulmonary artery
Abdominal aorta
Renal artery
Renal vein
Iliac arteries
Iliac veins
Femoral artery
Anterior tibial artery
Posterior tibial artery

Full body view of the circulatory system

Oxygenated blood (red) flows through arteries,
deoxygenated blood (blue) flows through veins

represents a worsening of symptoms and more damage to the heart and other organs. This is why early detection is essential. Simply put, the later the condition is caught, the less chance there is of regaining the use of a healthy heart.

CHF is cumulative – that is, each stage adds symptoms to those already manifested in the earlier stages.

THE GREAT COVER-UP: THE ASYMPTOMATIC STAGE

In CHF's earliest stage, the heart's output is just beginning to lag behind the body's demands. The body is highly sensitive to this deficit and may use a number of coping mechanisms. Any or all of the following may come into play, depending on the cause or severity of the condition.

Hypertrophic Cardiomyopathy

Just like a weight lifter strengthens muscles with strenuous exercise, so can the muscles of the heart strengthen and thicken when the heart has to work against an increased load. This is called Hypertrophic Cardiomyopathy.

Most often it is the left ventricle that thickens, because it has the hardest job to do. The left ventricle must pump the blood through the body's 60,000 miles of arteries, arterioles, capillaries and veins. Normally the left ventricle can handle the job, but when it has to work against long-term high blood pressure, it begins to struggle, causing the heart muscle to thicken in an attempt to compensate.

This thickening of the heart muscle gives the heart the strength to compensate for the added load, because a bigger muscle means more pumping force. But as the heart muscle thickens it becomes stiff, losing its elasticity. Decreased flexibility can have a significant effect on the function of the heart.

Think of the heart muscle as a rubber band around the heart. The pumping cycle of the heart is made up of beats and rests, or tightening and stretching. In between each beat, the heart muscle relaxes. As the heart muscle relaxes, the pressure of the incoming blood expands the heart chambers, stretching the heart muscle. Then, when the heart beats, the heart muscle tightens, squeezing the blood out.

The heart's efficiency is directly related to flexibility. The loss of elasticity in the muscle prevents the heart from relaxing as fully as it did before the heart muscle thickened. The chambers expand less, pulling in less blood and pumping out less blood with each beat.

This stiffness also effects the pumping action. While the action of the heart may be more powerful with the thickening of the heart muscle, the heart actually contracts less than it did, making each beat less efficient.

In addition, the blood needed to feed the enlarged area increases, placing more demands on a failing system.

Dilated Cardiomyopathy

Dilated Cardiomyopathy is the enlargement of the heart chambers. The muscles of the heart stretch more than normal at each rest, increasing the volume of the chambers and strength of the contractions.

The increase in heart chamber volume helps to pump more blood. For example, if you have an 8 ounce squeeze bottle that pumps 50 percent out with each squeeze, you release 4 ounces with each motion. But, if the bottle enlarged to hold 12 ounces, 50 percent would be 6 ounces or 2 ounces more for each squeeze.

Increasing the chambers' size also helps the heart to pump more strongly. Just like you would pull a bow back tighter to shoot an arrow farther, so does the heart muscle contract harder when it is stretched more.

But the long term stress of this stretching damages the elastic elements of the muscle fibers, reducing the muscle's elasticity and contracting strength over time. Eventually, the heart muscle weakens severely and the heart remains in this enlarged state. The chamber walls have been stretched thin and the enlarged heart can no longer pump as efficiently as it could at its original size.

Enlarged chambers can also lead to valve malfunction in more severe cases.

The flaps of the Mitral and Tricuspid valves in the left and right ventricles are attached to the sides of the chambers by muscular fibers called chordae tendinae. These valves

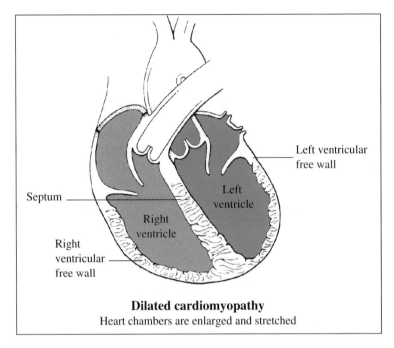

Left ventricular free wall

Septum

Left ventricle

Right ventricle

Right ventricular free wall

Dilated cardiomyopathy
Heart chambers are enlarged and stretched

prevent blood from flowing from the ventricles back into the atriums. The chordae tendinae help keep the valves from being blown open by the force of the contracting ventricles.

When the chambers enlarge to an abnormal size, they can pull the chordae tendinae, holding the valves partially open and causing some of the blood in the contracting ventricle to flow back into the atrium instead of forward into the lungs or out into the body. This results in a much less efficient and less powerful pumping action.

The stretched muscle has a higher blood demand than a normal heart muscle, further taxing a weakened system.

Hormonal Response

The same mechanisms that come into play when people are under stress or performing a strenuous physical activity are called into service when the heart's production falls below the body's needs.

Alerted by the lack of sufficient blood flow, the sympathetic nervous system begins to produce epinephrine (adrenaline) and norepinephrine. These natural stimulants cause the heart to speed up and beat with more force.

Boosting the heart rate can compensate for a damaged heart, for a while. Eventually, the stress can damage the heart muscle and lead to rhythm problems.

The Kidney's Response

The kidneys monitor blood flow and pressure. When the output of the heart falls, the kidneys react to the drop in blood volume. To compensate for the loss of volume, the kidneys release renin, which combines with angiotensinogen to form angiotensin.

Angiotensin causes the retention of salt, and thereby water, increasing the volume of the blood in the body. The increased volume means there is more blood for the heart to pump and therefore more blood pushing on the walls of the veins and arteries, raising blood pressure.

Angiotensin also affects the arterioles. The arterioles are small branches off the arteries that funnel the blood down into the capillaries. Constricting or dilating the arterioles is one of the ways the body alters blood pressure.

When the arterioles are constricted, the pressure of the blood rises; when dilated, blood pressure falls. Angiotensin acts on the muscles of the arterioles, constricting them and raising blood pressure.

Both of these compensation mechanisms provide temporary relief. The increased blood volume helps stretch the heart chamber walls, resulting in a stronger contraction and assuring that every part of the body receives blood.

The increase in blood pressure has a direct effect on the workload of the heart. Often, the blood pressure-related compensation mechanisms worsen the condition. The heart enlarges to adapt to the extra load, ultimately damaging itself.

The effects of high blood pressure can be widespread. High blood pressure can damage the tissues of sensitive organs including the eyes, the kidneys, the brain and the heart itself.

In the beginning, congestive heart failure has no symptoms. There is no physical indication that the compensation mechanisms are at work. Even heavy physical exercise, such as running, lifting or shoveling will not bring out symptoms of the condition.

The body's defenses can mask the symptoms, lulling those developing CHF into a false sense of security. Unfortunately, this makes early detection of CHF more difficult.

As time goes by, these compensation mechanisms actually damage the heart, diminishing its efficiency, putting more stress on it and accelerating the progression of the condition. These compensation mechanisms can be as detrimental to the body as the original cause of the heart failure.

If congestive heart failure can be detected in the asymptomatic stage, before the compensation mechanisms have advanced too far, it can be slowed, stalled or in some cases completely alleviated.

LEFT VENTRICLE FAILURE

When the compensation mechanisms lose their effectiveness, one or both sides of the heart may experience a significant drop in pumping capability. When this occurs the side is said to have failed. Generally, heart failure begins in the left ventricle because it has the hardest job to do.

Both sides of the heart work in unison to circulate the blood through the body. The right side takes in blood from the body and pushes it into the lungs. From there it returns to the left side, which pushes it out into the body again.

Because both sides work together, the drop in pumping ability of one side causes a destructive imbalance. When the left side fails, the right side continues to pump normally. But because the left side is pumping much less powerfully, it acts as a plug, causing the blood to back up from the failing left side into the lungs, where the blood pools.

The lungs are made of a thin sponge-like material with thousands of tiny air sacs, called alveoli. Each alveoli is surrounded by tiny arteries. A microscopically thin membrane separates the alveoli from the capillaries and allows the blood cells to release carbon dioxide and pick up oxygen.

Blood is made up of two main ingredients: the blood cells and a liquid called plasma. Plasma, which is mostly made up of water, carries the blood cells through the body.

The high blood pressure caused by the backup of blood

forces plasma out of the capillaries and into the alveoli, which manifests itself as congestion in the lungs. This congestion can be felt as a dry cough, due to irritation of the air sacs, and shallow breathing (apnea).

One very unpleasant symptom is paroxysmal nocturnal dyspnea (PND). People who have it wake up feeling like they are suffocating or smothering. They sit up gasping for breath and often throw open a window seeking "fresh air." This symptom can be eased to an extent by sleeping in a semi-vertical position.

The pooling of fluid in the alveoli impairs the exchange of carbon dioxide and oxygen. The poor oxygenation of the blood affects all areas of the body.

With fluid in the lungs and impairment of respiration, there is more likelihood of developing pneumonia, bronchitis or another type of respiratory infection.

RIGHT VENTRICLE FAILURE

Finally, as an end result of the added stress of working against the failed left ventricle, the right side also fails.

With the heart's function now severely impaired and the blood not circulating properly, gravity takes over.

Just as blood pooled in the lungs with left-sided failure, blood now backs up in the body itself, settling in the abdomen and legs. The increased blood pressure squeezes plasma out of the blood into the surrounding tissue. This is called edema.

To determine whether an individual has edema, press one or two fingers firmly on an area close to the ankle for about 10 seconds. If the indentation remains once the fingers are removed, edema is present.

Swollen with fluid, the abdomen and lungs take up more room, causing the heart, lungs and other organs to literally compete for space in the body. Adequate space is vital for the heart and lungs, as they must have room to expand and contract. People with CHF often have even less space due to their enlarged heart.

Severe crowding of the organs can be felt as a heavy weight on the chest. People who have this sensation should see if it is caused by edema or is a problem within the lung itself such as pneumonia, as the symptoms can be similar.

The most devastating effect of total heart failure is the lack of adequate blood flow throughout the body. During this time, most if not all of the organs of the body are affected with increasing severity.

THE EFFECTS OF INADEQUATE BLOOD FLOW

While there are specific symptoms that help determine whether an individual has left- or right-sided failure, there are symptoms that can occur with either stage. These problems are caused by inadequate blood flow.

Kidneys

As blood flows through the body it removes wastes from the tissues. Every part of the body produces wastes. The blood carries these wastes away to dispose of them.

The kidneys are the primary filter of the blood. Like a car's oil filter removes the wastes and byproducts of the engine's work, so do kidneys remove wastes from the blood.

For the kidneys to work properly, there must be enough pressure to push the blood through the kidneys' filtering tissues. When circulation drops, the kidneys' ability to filter the blood also falls. Many of the toxins that would normally have been removed by the kidneys continue to circulate through the body.

The high concentration of toxins left in the blood means it can't remove new toxins from the cells throughout the body. The buildup of toxins acts as a poison, severely weakening the cells. As the condition advances, they die.

While renal capabilities may be greatly reduced during the day because of the pooling of blood, at night the opposite happens. When a person lies down, the effects of gravity are negated and the pooled blood starts to circulate in a more normal fashion through the kidneys. This is called Nocturia.

During nocturia, the kidneys start working overtime to remove toxins from the blood. Unfortunately, the side effect of this is frequent urination. People with nocturia relieve themselves six or more times a night. This makes getting a good night's sleep almost impossible.

Heart

The heart, like any other muscle, needs an adequate blood supply in order to function properly. The lack of sufficient blood means the heart muscle does not get the oxygen and nutrients it needs. This weakens the heart muscle's ability to contract.

Since it is literally the "heart" of the circulation system, even a small drop in the heart's productivity has a great effect on the body as a whole.

Brain

The absence of adequate blood flow, coupled with the lack of sleep that often accompanies CHF, can have a strong effect on brain function. Confusion, emotional instability and decreased short- and long-term memory can all be experienced. The severity of these symptoms can vary widely from day to day, even hour to hour.

This impairment can be very dangerous for CHF sufferers who care for themselves. Confusion and memory loss can lead to overdosing or underdosing on medications. Many medications prescribed for CHF have life-threatening side effects if doses are missed or exceeded.

Liver

Inadequate blood flow can cause fluid to collect in the liver tissue. The liver needs a steady supply of fresh blood to be healthy and productive. When the liver becomes engorged with pooled fluid, the swollen tissue is starved for fresh blood and begins to sicken. This is called hepatomegaly.

Eventually liver cells begin to die. Liver cells are arranged so blood flows through them like a strainer. When liver cells die, the liver tries to compensate for the lost cells by generating new ones. But these new cells do not grow like the original cells. Instead, the area becomes a fibrous scar that actually blocks normal blood flow through the liver. This is called cirrhosis (scarring) of the liver.

Since blood must flow through the liver for it to do its

job, the scarred areas result in lost liver capacity. Advanced cirrhosis leads to almost total liver failure.

Circulation is one of the areas most affected by cirrhosis. The scar tissue in the liver acts as a block, backing up the blood going into the kidneys and causing high blood pressure, which leads to edema in the abdomen and extremities. The edema raises blood pressure even more.

Cirrhosis can cause anemia, the loss of red blood cells. Red blood cells are the vehicle by which cells receive oxygen and nutrients. Anemia makes the already deficient circulatory system even worse. Because the liver produces some of the elements that are part of the clotting process, cirrhosis can also affect the blood's coagulation mechanism so the blood does not clot normally.

Cirrhosis can disrupt the regulation of the body's potassium level. Potassium is one of the main minerals that ensures proper heart rhythm. Without the proper amount, dangerous rhythm disturbances can develop.

Cirrhosis also can cause loss of appetite, indigestion, nausea, vomiting, diarrhea or constipation.

Muscles

In response to the decrease in fresh blood, the body shifts the bulk of the blood supply away from the muscles to those areas that are essential for life, such as the organs.

This takes away the oxygen and nutrients the muscles need to do their work. The first indication of this shift is greatly reduced endurance and a feeling of overall fatigue. This fatigue may be felt early in the course of the condition. As the condition advances, strength and stamina diminish.

The lack of adequate blood flow can progress to the point where the muscles are literally starving. Initially, the muscles respond by using up their energy reserves. When the reserves are gone, the muscle begins to feed on itself. This can be seen as substantial and rapid loss of muscle mass.

The loss of muscle mass can be masked by water retention. A person's body weight may actually increase during this time, but they are losing muscle strength to support that water weight.

In time, a vicious cycle develops as the other symptoms accompanying CHF discourage physical activity, accelerating the loss of strength and muscle mass.

Skin

Congestive heart failure can even affect the skin. The lack of blood can prompt the body to reduce the amount of blood flowing to the skin in order to use it for more vital organs.

As a result, the skin of CHF sufferers can grow dusky and cool. People with CHF often become highly sensitive to temperature and may feel cold even when wearing a heavy sweater, while those around them are warm wearing only shirt sleeves and shorts.

Skin is the largest organ in your body and should not be overlooked. Without proper blood flow, wounds can be slower to heal, increasing the potential for infections and skin problems.

Digestive System

The digestive system has a crucial job to do. Here, the food we eat turns into fuel to run our bodies. The stomach and intestines need blood to digest our food.

The stomach and intestines manufacture acid to break down the food into a form from which the nutrients can be extracted. Without a proper blood supply, they can't manufacture the acids necessary to break down the food completely. The undigested food just passes through without giving the body energy.

In the intestines, blood picks up nutrients to feed the rest of the body. Blood flows through the walls of the intestines, receiving nutrients that pass through the thin membranes from the digesting food. When blood flow is inadequate, it can't reach all areas of the intestines to get all the nutrients that are in the food.

This disruption of the body's digestion can manifest itself as indigestion, constipation and diarrhea.

THE CAUSES OF HEART FAILURE

C ongestive heart failure – the inability of the heart to keep pace with the demands of the body – is not a disease, but a condition. There are a variety of causes, ranging from hypertension to anemia, that may make the heart pump improperly or make the work it has to do harder.

It's important to determine the underlying cause of the CHF. By identifying the cause, you identify the proper course of treatment.

Often, CHF may be triggered by a combination of two or more causes such as hypertension and coronary artery disease. In these cases, it is important that each factor that contributes to CHF be addressed and treated.

Rhythm Disturbances

Just like a car sends an electrical charge to the spark plugs, igniting each chamber in a particular order to produce power, so do electrical impulses cause the heart chambers to contract in a certain order to pump blood.

To understand heart rhythm and how it can be disrupted, we have to learn how the heart's conduction system works.

The "spark" originates at the sinus node, a collection of cells located high in the right atrium. This is the "pacemaker" of the heart, controlling the frequency and strength of contractions.

From the sinus node, the charge flows through conducting cells to the left atrium muscle, causing it to contract, and then continues on to the right atrium muscle, which also contracts.

The electrical impulse then moves to the atrioventricular (AV) node, a collection of cells in the middle of the heart just above the ventricles. The AV node slows down the impulse so that the atriums have time to contract fully.

Released from the AV node, the impulse flows down the area in the middle of the heart separating the left and right ventricles. The cells that carry it are called the His-Parkinje system. The impulse flows down through these cells and out to the muscle cells of the ventricles, causing them to contract. This whole process takes only one quarter of a second.

For the heart to pump correctly, the impulse must be the correct frequency and strength and follow the correct path, reaching every muscle area at the right time and in the proper sequence.

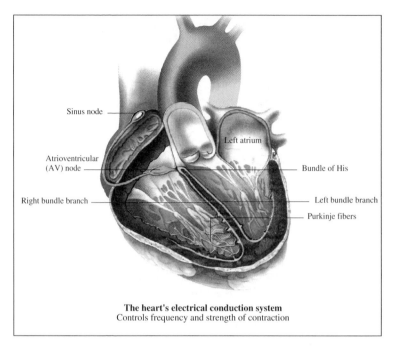

The heart's electrical conduction system
Controls frequency and strength of contraction

Because heart rhythm is so complex and many different areas are involved, a variety of factors can cause disturbances or arrhythmias. These factors fit into two main groups: physical problems and chemical problems.

Damage to the heart muscle, such as heart attack or an inflammation, can injure the cells that conduct the electrical impulse, weakening or blocking the flow of the impulses altogether.

Arrhythmias can even be caused by CHF itself. In the Asymptomatic stage, the stretching and straining of the heart muscle can damage the muscle cells, disrupting rhythm. By surrounding the heart with fluid and restricting space for movement, edema can also lead to arrhythmia.

The regulation of rhythm and the conduction of the impulses are primarily chemical processes. The formation of the impulses is an electrochemical process. Just like a car battery has to have the right mixture of acid to produce electricity, so does the sinus node need the right amount of chemicals.

Chemicals in and around the cells enable the impulses to flow from one cell to the next and contain the impulses to the conduction system. Without this chemical balance, impulses could be blocked, weakened or diffused through the heart.

One of the most common causes of arrhythmia are the chemicals in prescription drugs. There are thousands of drugs that list rhythm disturbances as a possible side effect – everything from allergy medications to diet pills. Diuretics can cause arrhythmias indirectly by removing potassium from the body.

Many common substances can affect heart rhythm, even drinking a cup of coffee or having a cigarette. Too much caffeine, alcohol or tobacco can cause arrhythmia. Conversely, inadequate amounts of magnesium and potassium in the body can also lead to arrhythmia.

The two basic forms of arrhythmias are Bradycardia and Tachycardia. Bradycardia basically means the heart is beating slower than it is supposed to, while Tachycardia means it is beating faster than it should.

There are three basic kinds of Bradycardia, based on which area of the conduction system is at fault. These areas are the nervous system, the sinus node and the heart's conduction system around the AV node.

The central nervous system monitors the entire body. It determines what the needs are and tells the sinus node to speed up or slow down. When the central nervous system malfunctions, it tells the sinus node to slow down too much or stop altogether. The heart can stop completely for 5 to 10 seconds, or even longer. Mild Bradycardia of this type can cause faintness or fatigue, while a severe case can be deadly.

There are many factors that can cause the central nervous system to malfunction ranging from a tight necktie to low blood pressure.

Called the "Pacemaker," the sinus node is where the impulses originate. When this area malfunctions, it is called "sick sinus" syndrome.

There is a relatively easy way to determine if someone has "sick sinus" syndrome: when the sinus isn't causing the heart to beat too slow, it's speeding it up. This alternation of slow and fast beats is often separated by pauses of up to a few seconds in length. The overall effect is faintness, nausea and fatigue.

Treating this problem can be difficult because both the

slow and fast impulses must be controlled. A pacemaker can be used to speed up the slow beats, but when the sinus node tries to beat fast it can disrupt the rhythm again.

When the conduction system fails, it is often called an AV block because the impulses are usually stalled in the area around the AV node. This type of problem stops the impulses trying to go down through the AV node and into the ventricles. The loss of these impulses causes skipped beats.

There are three degrees of AV block. First degree is very mild – sometimes there are no symptoms. It may only be found on an electrocardiogram test. Second degree is more severe. It is marked by the intermittent blocking of impulses, resulting in skipped or slowed beats.

Third degree, often called "Complete heart block," is the total blockage of impulses. While the heart may continue to beat, this is very serious and necessitates a pacemaker as soon as possible.

Bradycardia can lead to heart failure if the heart falls behind and is unable to keep up with the body's demands.

There are two basic kinds of Tachycardia or rapid rhythm disturbance. The first is where the heart rate is too fast for the body's needs. This is usually caused by a malfunction of the nervous system or the sinus node. These fast heartbeats often feel like a skipped beat as the heart pumps before it has had time to fill with blood.

In the second type, the cardiac cells themselves create the electrical impulse that initiates a contraction. Usually this message originates from the sinus node, but during Tachycardia the cells in or above the ventricles create a charge. This causes the surrounding area to contract out of sequence, misfiring. The heart beat splits into two distinct separate rhythms.

The rate of contraction in these areas may be totally different than that of the rest of the heart. The misfiring rhythm can be as fast as 250 beats a minute, while the rest of the heart may be beating at 70 beats a minute.

A heart with Tachycardia is very inefficient. While all or part of the heart is pumping more rapidly than normal, it actually pumps less blood because the chambers have no blood in them when they pump these extra beats. This strain can cause heart failure.

Hypertension

Hypertension, or high blood pressure, is one of the largest causes or contributing causes of CHF. Over 60 million Americans have high blood pressure. Of people over 60, about 54 percent have high blood pressure. By age 70, the rate rises to 64 percent.

Called "the Silent Killer," the vast majority of people with high blood pressure have no idea that they have it. Generally there are no symptoms. Of those who know they have it, only 25 percent receive adequate treatment. The cause is unknown in 90 to 95 percent of all cases.

To understand how high blood pressure can cause congestive heart failure, we must take a closer look at the circulatory system.

The body has a 60,000 mile network of blood vessels made up mostly of capillaries. Less than the thickness of a single human hair, these tiny arteries are so small that blood cells move through one at a time.

This single file progression enables each cell to come in contact with the extremely thin walls of the capillaries through which it deposits oxygen and nutrients while removing carbon dioxide and wastes. But the cells do not just flow through. They must be pushed through at a rate that allows the surrounding area to receive sufficient nourishment. To do this takes pressure.

Blood, like any other liquid, wants to find its own level. It will pool at the lowest point possible. Just like rainwater runs down out of the mountains and pools in the valleys, so would the blood drain out of from the upper body and pool in the legs.

If blood were allowed to follow that natural course in our bodies, we would die. Since we spend most of our lives in the vertical position, the heart must work against gravity to circulate the blood. The highest part or our bodies is also the most important recipient of blood – the brain.

For the circulatory system to work correctly, the blood must be at a pressure great enough to counteract the effects of gravity and push the blood cells through the capillaries from head to toe.

The body uses a number of regulatory mechanisms to keep the blood pressure at a level high enough for circulation to work properly. It raises or lowers this pressure in response to demands placed on the body by stress or physical exertion. Since everybody is different, this ideal level varies slightly for each individual.

A malfunction of these mechanisms or an effect of some other force in the body can raise the blood pressure beyond this level.

There are two measurements for blood pressure: Systolic and Diastolic. Systolic is the amount of pressure exerted when the heart is contracting (highest) and Diastolic is the amount of pressure felt when the heart is resting between the beats (lowest). A sample blood pressure reading would look something like this: 130/85.

The medical community has set up guidelines outlining what they believe are healthy and unhealthy blood pressure levels. While it is not an absolute, it can give us a good idea of what creates too hard a workload for the heart and what level is comfortable.

Systolic	Level
Less than 130	Normal
130 to 139	High Normal
140 to 159	Mild Hypertension
160 to 179	Moderate Hypertension
180 to 209	Severe Hypertension
210 or Higher	Very Severe Hypertension

Diastolic	Level
Less than 85	Normal
85 to 89	High Normal
90 to 99	Mild Hypertension
100 to 109	Moderate Hypertension
110 to 119	Severe Hypertension
120 or higher	Very Severe Hypertension

Generally if the upper number is elevated, the lower number usually is as well. That is not always the case, however, and that is why the systolic and diastolic guidelines are separated.

One of the biggest fallacies is that the ideal systolic blood pressure is your age + 100. Ideally, your blood pressure should remain in the 130/80 range. The guidelines are effective regardless of age.

Blood pressure is a measure of how hard the heart is working. While a certain amount of blood pressure is necessary for proper circulation, excess blood pressure actually works against the heart.

When blood pressure is abnormally high, the heart must work considerably harder to circulate the blood. The strain of this extra load and the damage high blood pressure can do to the cells of the heart muscle itself can lead to congestive heart failure. A variety of other problems can also arise from high blood pressure, contributing to the formation and advancement of CHF.

High blood pressure is easy to diagnose – the test is quick and painless. There are many places to have blood pressure tested besides your doctor's office, such as fire stations and drug stores. Blood pressure should be checked several times a year, especially for those who are at risk for CHF.

While high blood pressure is one of the biggest causes of CHF, it is also one of the most avoidable. Almost all cases of high blood pressure can be controlled through the use of herbs, diet and exercise, or blood pressure medications. Any of these treatments is preferable to coping with heart failure.

Coronary Artery Disease

In cases of coronary artery disease, the arteries leading to the heart muscles become partially blocked by plaque. The formation and buildup of this plaque is called Atherosclerosis.

This partial blockage reduces the normal flow of blood to the heart muscles, starving them of the oxygen and nutrients they need to do their work. Atherosclerosis can trigger the compensation mechanisms which, ironically, result in the heart muscle needing more oxygen – oxygen it can't get through the narrowed arteries.

An Electrocardiogram (ECG) test can reveal atherosclerosis as this type of condition has its own unique "signature" on the readout.

In cases where there is no significant damage to the heart muscle from a heart attack or other antagonist, treatment may take the form of an Angioplasty or a bypass operation to clear the blocked arteries. This is one of the few areas where either of these operations may be beneficial to someone with CHF.

Past Heart Attack

During a heart attack (Myocardial Infarction), a part of the heart muscle is deprived of oxygen and dies. While the heart may continue to function and the person may recover enough to feel healthy again, the heart has been compromised by the loss of muscle.

The physical damage can be twofold. First, there is the loss of contracting strength due to the reduction in muscle. Secondly, the dead area becomes a hardened scar, stiffening the chamber walls so the heart cannot expand fully, reducing the volume of blood drawn in by the heart. Both effects reduce the pump's power and capacity.

In addition, the death of part of the heart muscle can disrupt the heart rhythm. See the section in this chapter on Rhythm for more information.

These days, more people are surviving heart attacks and the severity and damage are being reduced with the application of "clot-busting" drugs. However, congestive heart failure is more of a risk for heart attack victims now than it was 10 years ago. CHF is a condition that targets heart attack survivors and, ironically, there are more now than ever.

Acidosis Versus Atherosclerosis

There is an alternative theory to the American atherosclerotic theory of how heart attacks occur. This theory, widely known and accepted in Europe, has some compelling evidence behind it. It also answers the nagging question that plagues the American atherosclerotic theory: Namely, why do some people who have obviously suffered a heart attack not have blocked arteries?

Like many European researchers studying alternative heart therapies, Peter Schmidsberger, noted author and president of the German League for Prevention of Coronary Disease, asserted that far too much attention is focused on the coronary arteries themselves and too little is given to how the heart muscle itself receives blood.

In his 1990 presentation before the World Research Foundation Congress in Los Angeles, Schmidsberger compared circulation of the heart to the roadway system of a busy metropolitan area. Highways (the coronary arteries) surround the city (the heart). Inside the city (heart) there are thousands of smaller side streets (the capillaries). These smaller streets go everywhere, connecting up with other streets and highways.

The blockage of the coronary arteries is a gradual process. It takes years for the arteries to narrow to the point of being blocked completely. Schmidsberger contends that in the time it takes for this process to reach the advanced stage, most of the blood has already been diverted to the smaller pathways.

When part of the highway (artery) is closed down due to an accident (clot), the remaining traffic is diverted through city streets where the smaller pathways (capillaries) allow the traffic (blood) to get where it is needed.

Part of the problem, according to the European theory, is the viscosity or thickness of the blood. Just like the oil in a car is measured by viscosity, so can the blood be measured for thickness. The measure of blood thickness is called the hematocrit level. It is a ratio of how much of blood is solids (blood cells) to how much is liquid (plasma).

The European theory holds that most of the blood that actually gets to the heart muscle cells travels by those smaller pathways. When the blood is too thick, it can't flow down many of these narrower pathways and areas of the heart muscle become deprived of blood, decreasing the exchange of nutrients for wastes in the muscle cells.

The heart's own high blood pressure compensation mechanisms can also reduce this exchange of wastes for nutrients in the cells. Because the heart cannot generate more cells than it has when we are born, the heart must thicken or stretch the muscle cells when it thickens or enlarges. The added size or length of the cells makes it harder for them to absorb nutrients and oxygen and get rid of their byproducts.

Both of these factors, the thickening of the blood and the abnormal size and shape of the heart muscle cells, reduce the heart muscle cells' supply of oxygen and nutrients. But more importantly, they also decrease the removal of byproducts. These byproducts contain toxins, many of which are acidic.

According to the Europeans, this build-up of acid in the heart muscle cells is the real cause of heart attacks – not blockage of the coronary arteries. When the acidosis reaches a certain level it destroys the muscle cells, causing the area to die.

While the end result is the same as for the atherosclerotic theory, i.e. the death of cells in the effected area, the treatment is totally different.

European researchers believe the answer is to decrease the viscosity of the blood so that it circulates more freely through the capillaries.

The drug Strodival or Strophanthin is used to neutralize the acidity of the muscle cells and increase their ability to use the oxygen they receive more efficiently.

By thinning the blood and reducing its acidity, researchers hope to prevent further damage and, by increasing the efficiency of the heart, prevent congestive heart failure from developing.

Alcohol or Drug Abuse

For people with heavy alcohol or drug use, the substances act as a poison in the heart muscle, attacking and weakening it. Often these toxins work against other organs in the body, weakening the system as a whole, making the person even more susceptible to congestive heart failure.

People whose history of alcohol or drug abuse is reasonably short may experience full recovery, as the heart muscle strengthens and shrinks back to its normal size. Those who have a longer history of abuse may not be so fortunate.

Heart Valve Disease

Proper function of the valves is just as important as the action of the heart muscle itself. While the heart muscle contracts to push the blood out, the valves keep it going in the right direction.

There are two basic malfunctions of the valves. The valves can be stenosed or held open, or blood flow through the valves may be blocked. These problems can be caused by atherosclerosis, disease or a congenital defect.

When the valves malfunction, the heart muscle's contraction may just send the blood back where it came from instead of forward through the lungs or the body.

The strain of trying to compensate for a malfunctioning valve and the decreased output of the heart combine to cause heart failure.

Valves that are malfunctioning due to a congenital birth defect generally must be replaced, while valves that are malfunctioning due to the formation of plaque may respond to balloon valvuloplasty.

The compensation mechanisms of the heart itself – the enlarging of the heart – can cause irreparable damage by thickening so much that the muscle obstructs the flow of blood or keeps the valves from closing.

Inflammation of Heart Muscle

The heart muscle or the pericardial sack surrounding the heart may become inflamed because of viral infection or rheumatism.

This inflammation is a disruption and invasion of the cells. Initial symptoms may include tenderness and swelling. In its advanced stages, the inflammation can damage a significant number of the heart muscle cells.

If the inflammation is discovered and treated before permanent damage has been done to the heart muscle, people usually recover fully and suffer no ill effects.

If not, there may be considerable permanent damage to the heart muscle. This weakens the muscles' pumping action, decreasing its output and leading to congestive heart failure.

Idiopathic

When a doctor says someone's CHF is "idiopathic," they are literally saying that they don't know what caused it.

That shouldn't be good enough.

It is important that every effort be made to discover the cause of a person's CHF. Only when the cause is found can an effort be made towards treating the root of the problem, not just the symptoms. If one doctor cannot determine the cause, try another.

Some CHF sufferers never know the cause of their condition. You don't want to be one of them.

Uncommon Causes

Prescription drugs can contribute to heart failure. Many drugs have adverse side effects such as raising blood pressure or causing arrhythmias. Even drugs taken to treat one aspect of CHF can contribute to another. For example, many diuretics remove potassium from the body and the mineral deficiency can give rise to arrhythmias.

If you are taking any drugs, even over-the-counter medications, it's a good idea to familiarize yourself with the precautions and potential side effects.

Congestive heart failure can be an unwelcome problem for an already overburdened expectant mother. It is not known exactly why pregnancy can trigger CHF, but there are many added stresses, both physical and metabolic, that could contribute.

While most cases of CHF disappear after the birth of the baby, some do not – and the reasons are unknown.

Anemia can also trigger CHF. Anemia is a condition where the blood contains an inadequate amount of red blood cells. Without enough of these cells, the blood can't transport the normal amount of waste and nutrients. The lack of nutrients and buildup of wastes can, over time, lead to heart failure.

Anemia can be caused by a variety of problems ranging from malnutrition to spleen disorders. If the anemia is alleviated before permanent damage is done to the heart, full recovery is possible.

Congenital defects are physical problems that we have from birth. Birth defects that cause CHF are usually malformations of the valves or the heart chambers. The problem reduces the heart's pumping capacity, causing heart failure.

Usually, the malformation must be repaired or replaced surgically. If no permanent damage has occurred to the heart or other organs, a full recovery is possible after the defect has been corrected.

Heart failure is one of many problems people with AIDS may experience. AIDS breaks down the immune system, making them susceptible to a variety of diseases some of which can attack the heart muscle. Often, for people with AIDS, heart failure is of lesser concern.

Iron buildup can lead to heart failure in some cases. The body can have excessive amounts of iron either due to numerous blood transfusions or an inability to process the iron contained in a normal diet. Excess iron builds up in the tissues of the heart, stiffening the muscle and preventing it from expanding and contracting as much as it should, triggering CHF.

Sometimes surplus iron can be leached out by removing blood from the body. Iron is one of the main components the body uses to make blood.

Basically, anything that can weaken or damage the heart can cause or contribute to heart failure. If the problem causing the CHF can be treated before permanent damage occurs, complete recovery is possible.

MEDICAL APPROACHES TO HEART FAILURE

Some drugs have been appropriately called 'wonder drugs' in that one wonders what they'll do next.

-ANNALS OF INTERNAL MEDICINE

HEART PERFORMANCE YARDSTICKS

These diagnostic tools provide a means to judge how each individual's heart "measures up" against the average healthy heart.

Cardiac Output

Referred to by doctors simply as CO, Cardiac Output is the amount of blood the heart pumps in a minute. It provides an overall measurement of how much blood the body is receiving from the action of the heart. It does not tell how the heart is doing this work or how much stress it is under while doing it.

The average Cardiac Output is about 5 quarts. CO can be measured using any of the following tests: coronary angiography, echocardiogram and nuclear scans.

Stroke Volume

Stroke Volume measures the amount of blood pumped out in one beat and shows how much work the heart does with each contraction.

This is important because while a person's Cardiac Output might appear normal, they may have an elevated heart rate that is compensating for the weakness of each contraction. Stroke Volume allows doctors to look closer at the heart's actual performance.

The average Stroke Volume is about 3 ounces. It can be measured using any of the following tests: coronary angiography, echocardiogram and nuclear scans.

Ejection Fraction

In one significant way, heart action is like breathing. When you exhale, you don't expel all of the air in your lungs. When the heart contracts, it does not expel all of the blood in the chambers. The ratio of the blood expelled versus the total volume of blood that was in the chamber before the contraction is called the Ejection Fraction.

The Ejection Fraction of a normal, healthy person is between 50 and 60 percent. Depending on how far the condition has progressed, people with CHF can range from the 40s down into the 20s with anything below that considered crisis stage.

A low ejection fraction can point to a stiff heart muscle unable to expand completely or a weakened heart muscle which cannot contract as strongly as it should. It can be measured using any of the following tests: coronary angiography, echocardiogram and nuclear scans.

The Cardiac Cycle

The process that the heart goes through with each heartbeat is called the cardiac cycle. The cycle is split into two parts, the systolic period and the diastolic period. The systolic period is the contraction of the heart muscles while the diastolic is the relaxing or expanding of the muscle.

When the heart is not contracting as well as it should, it is called systolic failure. When the heart is not expanding or relaxing properly, it is called diastolic CHF. Each type points to a different circulatory problem and necessitates a particular form of treatment.

The type of CHF a person has can be found using one or more of the following tests: electrocardiogram, coronary angiography, nuclear scans and echocardiogram.

Enlargement

Unless you're a professional athlete, any enlargement of the heart is a bad sign. It enlarges because, in its normal state, it can't keep up with the body's demands. Both Hypertrophic Cardiomyopathy (thickening of the heart muscle) and Dilated Cardiomyopathy (enlargement of the chambers) make the heart less efficient while increasing its need for oxygen and nutrients.

Usually the areas that are under the most stress, either because of damage or high workload, are the most enlarged. Therefore, the effected areas can point to the cause of CHF.

Enlargement of the left ventricle is most common and can indicate long-term high blood pressure. Increased size of other areas of the heart can be due to muscle damage, valve malfunction or lung problems.

The size and shape of a heart can be found using these tests: chest X-ray, electrocardiogram, coronary angiography, nuclear scans and echocardiogram.

Personal Patient Profile

The most important question of all is simply, "How do you feel?"

What symptoms you have, how severe they are and how long ago they appeared can indicate how far the condition has progressed, what might be causing it and what areas of the heart are most effected.

Keep track of the severity of the symptoms and try to gauge whether or not treatments are helping. Also watch for new symptoms that may be side effects of the treatment itself.

The most common symptoms of CHF are:

Fatigue – One of the biggest signs of heart failure is fatigue. While it's normal to have some decrease in strength and stamina as we age, people with CHF have an accelerated reduction in physical ability. In weeks or months they can lose what others lose over many years.

Often explained away as inadequate sleep, bad diet, lack of exercise or increased stress, this fatigue does not cause immediate alarm. Only after it has become debilitating is it recognized as unusual.

The chart on page 73 shows the Four Functional Stages of CHF, as determined by the New York Heart Association. There are examples given at each stage to help you determine which stage you or others may be experiencing.

Congestion – One of the most pervasive symptoms of CHF is congestion in the lungs, causing shortness of breath. The gathering of fluid in the lungs also irritates the air sacs and triggers coughing. These symptoms are often mistaken for a chest cold.

As the condition progresses, it can lead to severe sleeping problems as fluid moves into the lungs when the person is in a horizontal position.

People with this condition often wake up gasping for breath and feeling like they need some fresh air. They may start sleeping propped up on pillows or even in a chair.

Edema – Edema begins in the lower legs. It appears as increased size and smoothness around the ankle area. To test for edema, press firmly with two fingers by the ankle. If

Functional Classification of Persons with CHF:

Class 1
No limitation on physical activity even when engaging in heavy physical activities such as running, shoveling snow, playing tennis or chopping wood. Since stamina is unaffected, there are no symptoms such as fatigue or shortness of breath.

Class 2
Feeling fatigue or shortness of breath is likely during heavy physical activity and possible during normal activities such as climbing stairs or carrying groceries. No symptoms are apparent when sitting or lying down.

Class 3
More severe limitation of physical activity. May be unable to participate in strenuous activities such as running. Symptoms are likely to appear with even light physical exertion such as walking. Person is still comfortable while sitting or reclining.

Class 4
Discomfort possible at all times, including rest. Person feels fatigue, shortness of breath and other symptoms of CHF during any physical activity. Limited to light physical activities such as walking or standing with short bursts of moderate exertion such as climbing stairs.

a noticeable imprint remains after the fingers are removed, the person has edema.

As the condition progresses, edema also begins to form around the stomach and abdomen. The swelling in the feet and lower legs can become so severe that walking is painful.

Edema is a burden. In addition to adding weight to a body already weakened by CHF, edema raises blood pressure increasing the "load" on the heart. Fluid retention can also effect the liver, kidney and lungs. Fluid collecting in the chest cavity can push on the heart and collapse the lungs.

MEDICAL DIAGNOSTIC TESTS

Since the Asymptomatic stage of CHF has no symptoms, early detection relies on regular checkups.

The tests given during a routine physical should alert the medical staff that something is amiss. However, those who have a medical history that predisposes them to developing CHF, such as a past heart attack, high blood pressure or other heart damage, should alert the staff so additional tests can be scheduled if warranted.

While there are a great many tests that can be used to diagnose CHF, several of them are not commonly used because of their high cost, limited availability or incomplete information. The tests that are widely used are listed below.

Many of the tests listed, such as electrocardiogram, blood pressure and norepinephrine level, are low- or no-risk noninvasive procedures. "Noninvasive" means there is no cutting of the body and therefore, no risk of infection or other complications. These noninvasive tests should be requested first.

Blood Pressure

A quick, painless and risk-free procedure, the blood pressure test can help determine an individual's risk of developing heart failure. It can also indicate the presence of CHF, since elevated blood pressure is one of the main symptoms of the condition.

The measuring devices used are a sphygmomanometer and a stethoscope. The sphygmomanometer consists of an inflatable cuff, a gauge and a hand pump.

The subject is seated and the thick cuff is wrapped around their upper arm. The stethoscope is placed on the inner elbow near the cuff, pressing on a main artery.

The cuff is then inflated using the attached hand pump. The inflated cuff acts as a tourniquet, blocking the flow of blood through the arm. The air pressure is slowly released while the person administering the test listens for the first spurts of blood.

The point on the gauge where these first sounds are heard is called the systolic or upper reading. As the pressure in the cuff is lowered further, the sound becomes continuous as the circulation returns to normal. The point on the gauge where this occurs is called the diastolic or lower reading. The whole procedure takes about a minute.

Electrocardiogram

The Electrocardiogram or ECG (also called EKG) can reveal a variety of information about heart function. It can indicate rhythm disturbances, past heart attack or other damage to the heart muscle, inadequate blood supply to the heart, congenital heart defects, thickening of the heart muscle or enlargement of the chambers and even high or low potassium and calcium levels.

The test is safe, easy and painless. Sensitive electrodes are attached to various points on the chest. The electrodes monitor the electrical activity of the heart as it beats. This electrical activity is represented as a moving line with one heartbeat seen as a series of waves. Each part of the heartbeat can then be broken down and analyzed.

There is no risk in a conventional or resting ECG. The disadvantage is that the test is not infallible and should be used in conjunction with other tests.

24-Hour Holter ECG

Used primarily to track occasional rhythm disturbances, the Holter ECG records the electronic activity of the patient's heart as they go about their daily routine.

The patient carries the recorder, which is about the size of a camera case, with them for what is usually a 24-hour period. A series of sensors are attached to the person's skin under their clothes.

Holter ECG is used if arrhythmias are suspected but have not shown up in ECG tests in the doctor's office, or to determine the frequency of diagnosed arrhythmias. It shows how the person's heart handles the stresses of everyday life.

There is no risk in this procedure. The only disadvantage is the inconvenience of being tied to a recorder for a solid 24-hour period.

Echocardiogram

This non-invasive procedure uses the same technology as depth finders and fish locators – in a much more sophisticated form. Ultrasound, tones too high to be heard by humans, also allows expectant mothers a view of their developing fetus. For this procedure, it has been adapted to show the heart in action.

Ultrasound waves are emitted by a transducer – a combination speaker and microphone. The waves enter the body and bounce off the heart muscle and the valves. The transducer picks up the returning echoes and sends the data to a computer. The computer turns it into a visible image of the heart at work.

There are many different types of echocardiograms, each one showing the heart in different ways and giving different types of information about the heart. Echocardiograms can show the size and structure of the heart, the presence of valve problems, pumping strength deficiencies and abnormal blood flow.

Since it is non-invasive, an echocardiogram is risk free. The disadvantage is that 10-15 percent of echocardiograms have faulty readings and they are not recommended for obese or broad-chested patients. Because of this, an echocardiogram should be used in combination with other tests to form an accurate picture of the heart.

Chest X-ray

A chest X-ray is a picture of the chest cavity. An X-ray gun is aimed at the person's chest. The gun "shoots" X-rays through the body onto a special film.

A chest X-ray can show the condition of the lungs as well as the overall size and shape of the heart. It can also reveal the buildup of water (congestion) around the heart or in the lungs due to heart failure.

X-ray tests are non-invasive. The main risk involved in the procedure is that of developing cancer due to radiation exposure. This risk is negligible due to the small dose of radiation received from each X-ray.

Stress Hormone Test

When the body senses a drop in blood flow, the autonomic nervous system (the part of the brain that monitors body functions) causes norepinephrine and epinephrine to be manufactured. These are forms of adrenaline. They act on the heart, causing it to pump harder and faster.

The level of these two substances can be found using a blood test. By measuring this level, doctors can determine how much stress the heart is under. Generally, if the level is low, then the heart is functioning normally. If it is substantially elevated, the heart is working harder than normal.

This test can show if the heart is under abnormal stress. What it doesn't show is why. It is merely used to confirm that the heart is laboring.

Since it is primarily a laboratory test, a norepinephrine level test can be run as part of normal blood work. All that is involved is taking a blood sample.

Stress Tests

Not to be confused with the norepinephrine level test, stress tests are often given in conjunction with another test, such as ECG, nuclear scan or an angiogram.

Often, abnormalities in the pumping action of the heart that haven't shown up in normal tests will show up when the heart is under stress.

To simulate stress, the subject is made to walk on a treadmill or pedal a bicycle while they are being monitored for any physiological changes. Usually the stress test is performed for a 15 minute period, with a reading taken every 2½ minutes. Often subjects reach the limit of their endurance before the end of the test.

Due to this strain, there is a possibility of the test itself causing stress-related illnesses or injuries such as angina or even a heart attack.

Cardiac Catheterization

All of the following procedures use some form of cardiac catheterization.

A catheter is a long, flexible tube that is about as thick

as a piece of spaghetti. It can come with a variety of different devices on the tip, depending on the type of test being performed.

In all types of cardiac catheterization, the catheter is inserted in a vein or artery, either in the arm or groin area, and threaded to the heart.

Cardiac catheterization carries a certain amount of risk. The catheter can damage the arteries or veins and even the heart itself. It can cause clots to form, increasing the possibility of a heart attack. Problems at the site of the insertion of the catheter can include: excessive bleeding, bruising, blockage and infection.

The contrast mediums or inky substances released into the body to make the area being studied visible, can cause an allergic reaction in some cases. Reactions can range from nausea to serious disruption of heart action. Often drugs used to counteract allergic reactions are kept on hand near the operating team.

Cardiac catheterizations have a one-tenth of 1 percent mortality rate and 3 to 4 percent of the patients experience side effects or adverse reactions to the tests.

Nuclear Scans

While X-rays work by sending a stream of radiation into the body, nuclear scans work by introducing radiation into the bloodstream which gives off emissions that are translated into images by a special camera.

There are many different types of nuclear scans, but the basic operation is the same. Radioactive material is combined with the patient's blood and injected into the blood stream near the heart with a catheter.

Often this is done in conjunction with a stress test. A stress test is designed to place the patient's body under a certain amount of physical stress. For nuclear scans, the patient is usually pedaling a stationary bicycle during the test. Images are taken at rest and then at each level of increased exertion until the patient is too exhausted to continue.

Nuclear scans can yield a variety of information such as ejection fraction, the condition of the coronary arteries, the amount of blood reaching the heart muscle, the size of the heart chambers, ventricular function and more.

Different tests are used to gather different kinds of information. For example, a Thallium scan is used to measure the blood flow to the heart muscle, while a MUGA is used to learn the exact size and functioning capacity of the left ventricle.

Some nuclear scans are combined with the use of special cameras in a technique called Computerized Tomography or CAT scanning. This technique uses a series of cameras arranged in a vertical ring with the patient's body in the middle. The cameras rotate around the patient and, with the aid of a computer, create a three-dimensional image of the patient's heart at work.

One example of this type of test is a Positron Emissions Tomography or PET test. This test is used to show the metabolic processes of the heart muscle, giving insight into how much oxygen and nutrients the heart muscle receives and how efficiently it is used. This can provide valuable information about the overall condition of the heart muscle. However, the PET test is still quite expensive and not widely used.

Nuclear tests combine the risks of catheterization with those of a stress test. In addition, there is the risk of cancer from the radioactive materials used.

Biopsy

In a heart biopsy, a small sample of the heart muscle is taken from the patient and examined in a lab. In order to get that sample, a special catheter fitted with a set of jaws must be used.

The catheter is threaded through the vein into the right ventricle of the heart. The tip of the catheter is pressed up against the side of the heart chamber. The jaws are then closed, literally taking a small "bite" out of the heart muscle. The catheter is then removed and the sample is analyzed. Often numerous samples must be taken to have enough material for the lab work.

A biopsy is useful when trying to determine the nature or cause of inflammation of the heart muscle. By taking a small sample of the muscle itself, it can be analyzed to determine what foreign agents, such as a virus, may be present.

The disadvantages of this procedure include the risks involved in catheterization, compounded by having the catheter removed and inserted numerous times to get additional samples.

The "bites" taken out of the heart wall do not appear to cause problems, although a "bite" taken in the wrong place could damage the heart or valve.

Electrophysiology

This test is used to determine the cause of a heart arrhythmia. It works by measuring the flow of electrical impulses through the heart.

Electrical impulses cause the heart muscles to contract. When, where and how strong these impulses are determine the time, place and force of heart muscle contractions. The heart has a built-in conduction system that channels these impulses where they need to go. Electrophysiology tests this conduction system.

To perform the test, an electrode-tipped catheter is inserted into the heart. The electrode senses the flow of electrons through the heart walls. Doctors use this to make a "map" of the flow and determine which areas are not allowing electrons to pass correctly.

This test can also be used to induce an arrhythmia, either to determine how an occasional rhythm disturbance occurs or to see if a new drug is effective. Often three or four catheters may be used at the same time to create and measure the flow of electrons.

A potentially dangerous procedure, Electrophysiology includes the risks involved in catheterization and adds the risk of arrhythmias and even cardiac arrest due to the induction of arrhythmias.

TREATMENT OF CONGESTIVE HEART FAILURE

In treating someone who has CHF, there are two basic areas to be concerned with: enhancing the heart's capability to do more work and making the work the heart has to do easier. Making these two ends meet is the whole goal of drug treatment.

Treating Heart Failure by Prescription

Contracting strength and rhythm: Digitalis

Generic Name	Trade name
Deslanoside	Cedilanid-D
Digitoxin	Crystodigin
Lanoxin	Digoxin

Derived from the Foxglove plant, Digitalis has been in use for over 200 years for a variety of ailments.

Digitalis binds with the muscle cell receptors that regulate sodium and potassium levels. These levels determine the amount of calcium reaching the heart muscle. Increasing the amount of calcium stimulates muscle contractions, enhancing the force of the heartbeat and boosting the amount of blood pumped out with each beat.

By strengthening the heart's action, Digitalis directly counteracts many of the symptoms of heart failure such as edema and fatigue. It is one of the most common drugs prescribed for people with CHF. Digitalis also regulates the speed and rate of release of electrical impulses through the heart muscle, which helps to control arrhythmias.

Cautions and Side Effects: A potentially lethal problem with Digitalis is the possibility of overdose. This can occur either through an unintentional overdose by the patient or by inadequate monitoring of the level of the drug in the body.

Digitalis builds up in the heart faster than the body can get rid of it. Over time, the level of Digitalis in the body can reach toxic proportions. Up to 30 percent of hospital patients taking Digitalis are found to have some degree of toxicity.

Initial symptoms of overdose include loss of appetite, blurred vision, nausea, vomiting and diarrhea. As the overdose builds, the patient experiences headaches, weakness, apathy and arrhythmias that gradually worsen, eventually causing death.

The problem is common and serious enough that there is a whole class of drugs that are available for use in case of such an overdose.

The danger is that the person may not get attention in time. This can be a distinct possibility for those in the later stages of CHF who care for themselves. The confusion and memory impairment that can occur in the later stages makes them highly susceptible to unintentional overdose.

People who have had significant heart muscle damage due to a heart attack have an increased risk of sudden death while taking Digitalis.

When coupled with a potassium-depleting diuretic, the effects of Digitalis can combine with the potassium deficiency to cause dangerous arrhythmias. This is a real danger for people with CHF, as these two types of drugs are often prescribed together.

Other commonly prescribed drugs for CHF that may interact with Digitalis are Quinidine and Verapamil, both anti-arrhythmics. The rhythm-depressing effect of Digitalis can combine with either one of these drugs to cause severe arrhythmias with the possibility of the heart stopping altogether.

Other commonly used drugs Digitalis can interact with are antacids, the antibiotic Erythromyacin and even foods such as oat bran.

For Angina: Nitrates

Generic Name	Trade Name
Isosorbide mononitrate	Imdur, Ismo, Isordil
Nitroglycerin	Minitran, Deponit, Nitro-Bid, Nitro-Dur, Nitrogard, Nitrol Ointment, Nitroglycerin SR, Nitolingual Spray, Nitrong, Nitrostat, Transderm-Nitro

These are the drugs of choice for the acute onset of angina – chest pain caused by a lack of blood to the heart muscle. They are all based on Nitroglycerin, a powerful artery dilator.

Nitroglycerin relaxes the smooth muscles of the arteries, causing them to expand. This dilation makes blood flow easier, reducing the workload on the heart. Nitroglycerin also increases the amount of blood reaching the heart muscle by dilating the coronary arteries.

Cautions and Side Effects: The sudden drop in blood pressure can momentarily deprive the brain of blood, causing dizziness or even fainting. Therefore, it is best to sit down if at all possible when taking the drug.

Other side effects include dizziness, headache or feeling flushed. With the sharp drop in blood pressure, the body could react by sending a message to the heart to pump rapidly. This response, called Reflex Tachycardia, could worsen the symptoms by stressing the heart.

Care must be used when storing and carrying Nitroglycerin. If the pills are subjected to excess heat or moisture, they can lose their effectiveness. Also, with repeated use, the duration of relief can diminish.

For Rhythm: Anti-arrhythmics

Generic Name	Trade Name
Moricizine	Ethmozine
Disoprymide	Norpace, Rhythmodan, Promine
Procainamide	Pronestyl
Quinidine	Duraquin, Quinaglute Quinalan, Quinate, Cardioquin,
Lidocaine	Xylocaine HCI, Xylocard
Mexiletine	Mexitil
Phenytoin	Dilantin
Tocainamide	Tonocard
Encainide	Enkaid
Flecainide	Tambocor
Propafenone	Rythmol
Acebutolol	Monitran, Sectral
Esmolol	Brevibloc
Propranolol	Inderal, Detensol
Amiodarone	Cordarone
Bretylium	Bretylol, Bretylate
Verapamil	Calan, Isoptin

Heart rhythm is so complex, no one drug can treat all the possible rhythm problems. The drugs used for arrhythmias are prescribed according to what area of the heart is experiencing problems (ventricles or atriums) and what change doctors believe will stop the arrhythmias.

There are a number of drugs that are often used for rhythm problems but actually are designed for other uses; such as Verapamil – a calcium channel blocker; beta-blockers Acebutolol, Esmolol and Propranolol; and Digitalis. See the respective sections on these classes for more specific information on how each drug works and their cautions and side effects.

Virtually all anti-arrhythmic drugs work to slow or lessen some part of the heart's rhythm. They do this by changing the concentration of electrolytes in the heart muscle. Electrolytes are minerals, such as calcium and potassium, that are used in the heart muscle to conduct the energy that makes the muscle contract.

Cautions and Side Effects: Any of these drugs can cause the formation of new arrhythmias. Because these drugs depress the action of the heart, the body can receive an insufficient supply of blood, impairing a variety of functions. They can also cause CHF or worsen the symptoms of those with CHF.

While these drugs may reduce or eliminate arrhythmias, some of them carry more hazards than they cure. Studies show taking Quinidine increases the likelihood of death over not using any drug at all.

Excessive deaths have also been reported in the use of other common Class I anti-arrhythmic drugs including Tambocor (Flecainide), Enkaid (Encainide), Ethmozine (Moricizine) and Mexitil (Mexiletine). After two studies performed in 1989 and 1991 by the National Heart, Lung and Blood Institute revealed the dangers of Tambocor, Enkaid and Ethmozine; only Enkaid (Encainide) was pulled off the market by the manufacturer.

The side effects of each anti-arrhythmic drug can vary. Many are serious and can include liver damage, lupus, convulsions, gastrointestinal problems, fever and nausea.

Some of these drugs can build to toxicity in the heart and lungs, which can be fatal. Neurotoxicity (a toxic accumulation in the nerves of the heart) can occur in up to 40 percent of patients with weakness and numbness as the main indicators.

Some of these drugs can take a long time to leave the body. Many can still be detected up to nine months from the time they are discontinued.

For Acidosis: Strodival

Generic Name	Trade Name
Strodival	G-Strophanthin

Price: $20.00 (U.S.) per 100 capsules

A whole distinct theory about the cause of heart attacks has risen from the positive effects of this drug. That theory holds that heart attacks are not caused by the sudden formation of a clot in the coronary arteries but by a buildup of acid in the heart muscle tissues. Strodival counteracts the buildup of acid in the muscle tissues, thereby allowing the tissues to get the oxygen and nutrients they need to function properly.

Strodival is classed as a general "heart tonic" in Europe, where it is used for a variety of problems including angina, heart attack and CHF. It has been found to be highly effective against angina in double blind tests – 81 percent of one test group was found to have significant relief from the symptoms of angina after taking the drug.

Strodival has also been very effective in stopping heart attacks in progress. Researchers found a full 85 percent of patients had relief from heart attack symptoms shortly after taking Strodival.

Because of its positive effects on oxygen and nutrient supply in heart muscles, the drug is thought to be well-suited for CHF patients, especially those with coronary artery disease.

Cautions and Side Effects: Since this drug is not widely used in the United States, we do not have a wealth of information on its potential problems. However, information from Europe, where the drug has been used widely for decades, show its side effects to be virtually nonexistent.

For more information on the drug and this alternative theory of heart problems, contact:

World Research Foundation
15300 Ventura Blvd., Suite 405
Sherman Oaks, CA 91403
(818) 907-5483

The drug can be purchased by contacting the pharmaceutical company that manufactures it. To import the drug, you must have a doctor's written prescription order and the drug must be sent directly to the patient for their sole use. Write, phone or fax inquiries to:

Herbert Pharma Gmbh
Am Wolfsfeld 17
65191 Wiesbaden, Germany
Tel: 0611-50-07-25
Fax: 0611-50-38-89

HIGH BLOOD PRESSURE DRUGS

Beta-Blockers

Generic Name	Trade Name
Timolol	Blocadren
Nadolol	Corgard
Propranolol	Inderol
Metoprolol	Lorpressor
Labetalol	Normodyne
Acebutolol	Sectral
Atenolol	Tenormin
Labetalol	Trandate
Pindolol	Visken

One of the body's reactions to the failing heart is to tell it to pump harder and faster. Beta-blockers block the heart's beta receptors from receiving this command. The heart then returns to its normal strength and pace. Because the heart isn't pushing as hard, the blood pressure drops.

Also, because the heart isn't pumping as hard, it needs less oxygen to function, relieving angina.

Cautions and Side Effects: Beta-blockers can cause fatigue, lightheadedness, impotence, depression, hallucinations, confusion or nightmares, generally due to the decreased cardiac output.

They can trigger breathing difficulties in people who have asthma, emphysema, bronchitis or other respiratory problems. This can be a significant problem for people with heart failure since fluid has already been building up in the lungs. Since beta-blockers can trigger or worsen these conditions, make sure your doctor knows about them.

Most importantly, beta-blockers are not recommended for the later stages of CHF because they diminish the performance of an already inadequate heart. This can worsen the symptoms and accelerate CHF.

Diuretics (Loop)

Generic Name	Trade Name
Bumetanide	Bumex
Ethacrynic acid	Edecrin
Furosemide	Lasix, Myrosemide, Novosemide, Uritol

Diuretics (Thiazide)

Generic Name	Trade Name
Bendroflumethiazide	Naturetin
Benzthiazide	Exna, Hydrex
Chlorothiazide	Diuril
Cyclothiazide	Anhydron
Hydrochlorothiazide	Diuchlor-H, Esidrix, HydroDIURIL, Novohydrazide, Oretic, Urozide, Maxzide
Hydroflumethiazide	Diucardin, Saluron
Methylclothiazide	Aquatensen, Diuretic, Enduron
Polythiazide	Renese
Trichlormethiazide	Metahydrin, Naqua, Trichlorex

Diuretics (Potassium-Sparing)

Generic Name	Trade Name
Amiloride	Midamor
Spironolactone	Aldactone, Novospiroton
Triamterene	Dyrenium

Easily the most widely used class of high blood pressure drugs, diuretics are commonly called "water pills." They work by causing the kidneys to excrete sodium in the urine. Sodium causes the body to retain water. When the level of sodium in the body drops, the kidneys begin taking more water out of the body and eliminating it through the urine.

There are three main types of diuretics, each classed by which area of the kidneys they work on. Thiazide diuretics work in the tubules, where urine is transported out of the kidneys. They are the most common type and are generally fairly effective.

Loop diuretics are more potent. They work in an area called the Loop of Henle. They are often used when Thiazide diuretics are insufficient or when the kidneys are not functioning properly.

Potassium-sparing diuretics work in the area of the kidney where potassium is excreted. They are used for those who are susceptible to the ill effects of potassium deficiency.

Cautions and Side Effects: The most significant problem with diuretics is the possibility of potassium deficiency. Potassium is necessary for proper functioning of many systems of the body – especially the heart. The mineral controls the impulses which tell the heart muscles to contract. Serious rhythm disturbances can occur without sufficient potassium. Digitalis exacerbates these arrhythmias.

Potassium supplements may not fully address the problem. Even Potassium-sparing diuretics can deplete potassium. Long term use of diuretics can cause severe electrolyte imbalances. Symptoms of electrolyte imbalance include weakness, lethargy, dizziness, vomiting and confusion.

Loop diuretics can work so well as to cause dehydration, lowering the volume of the blood so much that the circulatory system cannot function. Milder forms of this dehydration can cause clots to form. All forms of diuretics can cause hypotension or low blood pressure, which can lead to lethargy, impotence, dizziness or loss of consciousness.

Diuretics are known to interact with other circulatory drugs. When combined with Coumadin, the clotting ability of blood may drop to dangerous levels. Digitalis users are very susceptible to rhythm disruption. When diuretics are combined with an artery-dilator such as Nitroglycerin, the effects can be life threatening as the blood pressure can drop so low that it causes circulatory failure.

Calcium Channel Blockers

Generic Name	Trade Name
Bepridil	Vascor
Dilitiazem	Cardizem
Nicardipine	Cardene
Nifedipine	Procardia, Adalat, Apo-Nifed
Verapamil	Calan, Isoptin

A relatively new type of blood pressure drug, calcium channel blockers work as vasodilators. They block calcium to the cells that control the size of the blood vessels.

Calcium is needed by the muscles in the blood vessels to constrict. Deprived of calcium, the muscles relax, opening or dilating the blood vessels and lowering blood pressure.

One type of calcium channel blocker called Verapamil is also effective with some arrhythmias, and can be prescribed for that purpose as well.

Cautions and Side Effects: Calcium channel blockers are still relatively new, so not much is known about long-term effects. Headaches and constipation are two recognized side effects.

Calcium channel blockers interact with some major circulatory drugs. They can cause arrhythmias or hypertension if given with beta-blockers, and may allow Digitalis and Quinidine (an anti-arrhythmatic drug) to reach toxic levels in the body by blocking the liver from removing them.

Because of the lowered blood pressure, people taking this drug should avoid standing up quickly, as they may experience dizziness and even loss of consciousness as the brain is momentarily deprived of blood.

One type of calcium channel blocker has been found to be significantly more dangerous than the others. Procardia or Adalat (generic name Nipedipine) has been found to cause nearly twice the number of deaths as other comparable drugs over a period of five years. Federal health officials have warned that the drug should be used with caution, if at all.

ACE Inhibitors

Generic Name	Trade Name
Benazepril	Lotensin
Captopril	Apo-Capto, Capoten
Enalapril maleate	Vasotec, Enalaprilat
Fosinopril	Monopril
Lisinopril	Prinivil, Zestril
Quinapril	Accupril
Ramipril	Altace

Enjoying widespread popularity, ACE inhibitors are now considered by many to be the "first line" in the offense against high blood pressure.

ACE inhibitors are also highly valuable in treating the condition of CHF as well. Recent tests have shown ACE inhibitors, if administered in the early stages of CHF, can slow the progression of left-sided heart failure.

Like Calcium channel blockers and Alpha-blockers, ACE Inhibitors are vasodilators. Angiotensin converting enzyme inhibitors, or ACE inhibitors as they are called, block the formation of angiotensin II in the body. Angiotensin II is a powerful vasoconstrictor and also causes the body to retain sodium and therefore fluid.

As the level of angiotensin II drops, the veins and arteries open, lowering blood pressure. ACE inhibitors are especially useful for CHF because they lower blood pressure and help to reduce edema.

Enalaprilat, an ACE inhibitor taken intravenously, is enjoying considerable success in treating end-stage CHF patients in hospital intensive care units, where it has proven effective in improving heart function and lowering blood pressure.

Cautions and Side Effects: ACE inhibitors can cause the body to retain too much potassium, resulting in a condition called hyperkalemia. Foods or drugs high in potassium can add to this problem. Just like too little potassium can cause heart problems, so can too much.

Hyperkalemia can cause depressed heart function. If left untreated, the condition can make the heart stop altogether. It is very important to have your potassium level checked regularly while using ACE inhibitors.

Minor side effects of ACE inhibitors include fatigue, nausea, vomiting, diarrhea, dizziness, skin rash, swelling and loss of sense of taste. Some develop a persistent dry cough that usually goes away when the drug is discontinued.

The drug can lower the white blood cell count, leaving the user susceptible to infections. Common symptoms of this can include fever, sore throat, chills and mouth sores.

An allergic reaction to ACE Inhibitors is also possible. This can be indicated by swelling in the face, hands, feet or mouth. Sudden difficulty in breathing or swallowing may occur. If it does, seek help immediately.

Angina or arrhythmias may arise from the use of ACE Inhibitors. Most often this only happens initially, but if it seems serious seek help.

The drug may depress the action of the kidney. If there

is an increase in body weight or edema, discontinue the drug and see your doctor.

ACE inhibitors can interact with some drugs used for treatment of CHF. The effects of ACE inhibitors are enhanced by beta-blockers, diuretics and alcohol. The danger from this is excessively lowered blood pressure resulting in dizziness, fainting and circulatory failure.

Nonsteroidal anti-inflammatory drugs such as Aspirin, Ibuprofen, Indocin, Naproxen, Toradol and many others can negate the effects of ACE inhibitors and cause salt and fluid retention.

Alpha-Blockers

Generic Name	Trade Name
Phenoxybenzamine	Dibenzylene
Phentolamine	Regitine
Prazosin	Minipress
Terazosin	Hytrin

One of the ways the body controls blood pressure is by controlling the size of the arteries. When the body determines that it is not receiving enough blood (as in CHF), it sends out a chemical signal to tell the arteries to constrict. This message is received in the arteries by the alpha receptors.

Alpha-blockers block the alpha receptors from telling the muscles of the arterioles to constrict. This causes the muscles to relax, expanding the arterioles which lowers blood pressure and lessens the workload on the heart.

Cautions and Side Effects: Due to lowered blood pressure, people taking this drug should avoid standing up quickly, as they may experience dizziness and even loss of consciousness as the brain is momentarily deprived of blood.

Other symptoms of lowered blood pressure can be pinpoint pupils, impotence and nasal congestion.

Anti-Coagulant (clotting) Drugs

Generic Name	Trade Name
Warfarin	Coumadin, Panwarfin, Warfilone, Sofarin

Commonly called "blood-thinners" this type of drug actually lowers the blood's ability to clot, slowing down the clotting process and making it less likely for unwanted clots to form.

Warfarin, often referred to under the trade name Coumadin, partially blocks the liver's absorption of vitamin K (named by the Germans for its role in the "Koagulation process"). This vitamin regulates the level of clotting agents in the blood.

As the level of vitamin K in the liver decreases, so does the level of these clotting factors in the blood and therefore blood takes longer to clot.

Cautions and Side Effects: Since the drug competes with vitamin K for space in the liver, the level of vitamin K in the body can greatly affect the time that it takes for the blood to clot. Vitamin K is manufactured in the intestines, but the main way of receiving it is through diet. Those taking Coumadin must be careful not to eat too much of foods high in vitamin K such as kale, spinach, broccoli, cauliflower, green tea, soybean oil and animal livers.

The drug is highly susceptible to interactions with other substances. Even common drugs such as alcohol, aspirin and Tylenol can increase or decrease the effectiveness of Coumadin. Significantly, drugs such as diuretics and anti-arrhythmics used by many CHF patients can also influence the effects of Coumadin.

The consequences of having a clotting ability that is too high or too low can be very serious. If blood clots too slowly, there is a very real possibility of bleeding to death. Even small cuts and scrapes can be life threatening. Large overdoses can cause internal bleeding and death. Coumadin is a central ingredient in many brands of rat and mouse poison. The rodents bleed to death from the overdose.

Excessive clotting can be life threatening by allowing clots to form in the blood stream, causing strokes, heart attacks and other circulatory problems.

Since the correct level is so important and because Coumadin is easily affected by so many factors, it's important to have a regular test of your blood's clotting ability. This test is called the "pro-thrombin time." It measures the time it takes for your blood to clot. Between tests, watch for early warning signs, such as excessive bruising and blood in urine or stools.

Aspirin

Generic Name	Trade Name
Aspirin	Anacin, Bufferin, Easprin, Empirin, Excedrin, Florinal, Gelpirin, Lortab, Norgesic, Percodan, Supac, Talwin, Zorprin, Soma Compound

Aspirin has been around for over one thousand years, but it is only lately that it has gained attention as an anti-clotting drug. Aspirin helps keep platelets from coming together to form a blood clot.

**Cautions and Side Effects**: The main problem with aspirin is overdose. Because the drug has been a household fixture for ages, it is not taken seriously. An overdose of aspirin can cause bleeding in the stomach and brain which can be fatal.

The amount of aspirin that is actually necessary to achieve the anti-clotting effect is surprisingly small – only 40 mg. a day. Taking more than that increases the risk of stomach irritation.

Oxygen

By inhaling an oxygen-rich blend of air, people with CHF can compensate for the decreased ability of the lungs to properly oxygenate the blood. Making the blood richer in oxygen takes a strain off the heart by reducing the demand of the body and giving the heart muscle itself an adequate supply of oxygen.

This is often a necessity for sleeping, as the capacity of the lungs falls greatly due to fluid collecting in the lungs when lying down. Oxygen can combat this drowning feeling, making a good night's sleep possible.

There are two main sources of oxygen available: oxygen tanks and machines. The tank is about 2½ feet long and 3 inches in diameter with a regulator, hose and face mask. The main advantage of the tank is a higher degree of portability because it fits into a small, wheeled hand dolly. For short term use, such as social outings, tiny hand-held tanks are also available.

The machine is about the size of a foot stool. It creates its own oxygen, therefore does not need constant refilling. Because of its size, the machines are generally stationary with an extra long supply hose so the user can move about.

Cautions and Side Effects: Despite the wheeled dolly, tanks can be cumbersome and heavy, especially for someone with CHF. Changing them can be a chore.

The tanks can run out, unlike the machines which, if they have electricity, can supply oxygen indefinitely. People using tanks often contract with a medical supply service to bring fresh tanks and remove the used ones.

Machines are not very portable, tying the user to the base of supply. A very real concern is a power outage. Without power, the machines cannot produce oxygen. Therefore, it is wise to keep oxygen tanks nearby – just in case.

Oxygen should be used only when necessary with the long term goal of weaning off use, if possible. Continual use of oxygen can mask the worsening of the condition.

It is common for people using oxygen to deteriorate since they are tethered to the machine and do not get the exercise they need to improve.

NEW DRUGS

One area where CHF is receiving the attention it deserves is in the pharmaceutical industry. There are a large number of drugs, some still in development and some soon to appear, which many hope will provide real alternatives to the often debilitating drugs of today. Here are a few that should be in the news and the pharmacies in the not so distant future:

Endothelin Blockers are a new class of drugs that works to block the function of Endothelin, a powerful regulator of blood flow and blood pressure. Still in the experimental stage, Endothelin Blockers could be an attractive alternative for people who cannot tolerate the current group of high blood pressure drugs.

Hypothalmic Inhibitory Factor (HIF) Drugs target HIF, a natural hormone found in the human body which regulates the "sodium pump," an enzyme found in all cells. Sodium determines the level of fluids in the body and is used for contraction by heart muscle cells. Researchers believe this could hold the key to regulation of blood pressure and heart muscle function, two big factors in CHF.

Bucindolol is a new type of beta-blocker, said to greatly improve the function of the left ventricle in people with CHF. It combines this beta-blocker action with a mild vasodilator effect to moderate blood pressure. Bucindolol is currently undergoing trials with people afflicted by CHF to determine if it significantly improves survival rates.

Sotalol is a new drug that combines the effects of different kinds of beta-blockers in one. Sotalol just became available in the U.S. in 1995. Because the drug works on multiple areas of heart function, it is an ideal anti-arrhythmic. Clinical tests have proven Sotalol to be more effective than comparable anti-arrhythmics in preventing arrhythmias.

Vesnarinone is a derivative of Quinolone, a drug that has been used for many years as an antibiotic to treat urinary tract infections. Recent research has found a new use for the drug as a stimulant of heart function.

Vesnarinone seems highly effective in stimulating the contraction of the heart muscle, resulting in increased circulation. In early tests, the drug was found to reduce heart failure mortality by up to 60 percent. Further clinical tests are being conducted to verify the drug's miraculous effects.

Since Vesnarinone has been on the market for some time, we know its main side effects. The drug can cause cartilage damage, especially in the young whose bones are still growing. Because of this, the drug is not prescribed for young people. More significantly the drug can affect the central nervous system, causing headache, dizziness, seizures and changes in vision. Those with a preexisting central nervous system disorder should not take the drug.

In addition, the drug can react with certain substances

such as sodium bicarbonate (baking soda) and antacids in the kidneys, causing a painful condition where urine crystallizes in the urinary tract. With careful attention to diet, this problem can be easily avoided.

CPC-111 works to stimulate the metabolism of the heart muscle cells during times of oxygen depravation. By doing this, CPC-111 minimizes damage to the muscle during times of stress. The reduced damage results in greater muscular strength, and therefore, better circulation. This drug is currently undergoing trials to verify its effectiveness.

Carvedilol is actually not a new drug – the drug has been approved by the FDA for treating high blood pressure, but it hasn't been made available to patients. New studies have shown a potentially beneficial role for the drug to play in the fight against CHF.

In a series of clinical trials of people suffering from CHF, Carvedilol seemed to reverse heart failure, cutting the number of deaths by two-thirds. Another study found the drug reduced the number of hospitalizations by 40 percent. The drug's chief side effect was dizziness.

Carvedilol is a new type of beta-blocker that does not have the negative effects on heart action of other beta-blockers. In addition, it also has a mild vasodilating effect, helping lower blood pressure further.

Carvedilol will soon be released under the brand name Coreg and marketed as a drug specifically for people with CHF.

SURGERIES FOR HEART FAILURE

Transplant

Heart Transplants are for people who have severe heart muscle or valve damage, but who are otherwise healthy. Transplant operations are generally seen as a procedure of last resort because of the risks involved.

The biggest problem with heart transplants is the shortage of available hearts. While over 15,000 people each year are candidates for the procedure, only 2,000 hearts are available. If the other 13,000 are lucky, they can survive until next year.

Potential recipients are put on a list with priority given to those whose hearts have failed completely. For the majority, it is a tense waiting game.

Once the heart is secured, the concern becomes surviving the surgery. Many die in the first three months from organ rejection and infection. Only 80 percent of heart recipients survive the first year. After that first critical year, the odds improve. About 70 percent survive 5 years and almost 50 percent survive 10 years. Some recipients have lived over 20 years.

Anti-rejection drugs are used to protect the new heart by suppressing the immune system's ability to function so it will not attack the heart as a foreign object in the body. This breaks down the body's natural immunity, leaving the recipient vulnerable to a variety of diseases and infections.

Anti-rejection drugs must be taken for the rest of the recipient's life. Common side effects include vulnerability to infection, liver and kidney impairment, high blood pressure, weight gain, diabetes, gallstones, joint damage and water retention.

The financial burden of a heart transplant can be enormous. Costs for the basic procedure and a short hospital stay can start around $80,000. But this may only be the beginning; with the possibility of complications and rejection, an extended stay in intensive care can run well over $200,000.

LVAD

An emerging alternative to transplant is the Left Ventricular Assist Device or LVAD. Originally developed to keep prospective heart recipients alive while they waited for a heart, the device has been refined to the point where it could offer a significant improvement in the quality of life for many people with severe CHF.

LVAD is much less radical and risky than a heart transplant. Instead of taking over the function of the whole heart it assists the left ventricle which has the biggest job and is therefore most likely to fail.

The device does not take over the circulation of blood

entirely. It takes 25 to 50 percent of the blood coming into the heart and pumps it out into the body. This allows the heart to still function normally while circulation is given a significant boost.

Early LVADs were large and cumbersome. Most of them actually had the whole pumping mechanism outside the body with two hoses inserted inside to circulate the blood. These external devices were prone to cause blood clots and were only used for short periods of time.

The newer devices are completely internal and only about the size of a plum. The internal LVADs enable the users to have almost unrestricted mobility.

As the design of the device steadily improved, so has its track record. The average time of use has grown from days and weeks to months and now is approaching a year. Some patients have used the device for over 400 days. The goal of current research is to create a device that will last up to five years.

Since an LVAD does not replace the heart, there is no fear of rejection and no need for the drugs transplant patients must rely on. For those stricken with an acute heart problem that is causing CHF, the device can allow their heart to rest and recover.

LVADs are just emerging from the experimental stage so the risks and side effects of the device are not fully documented. Two known problems are risk of infection and the formation of blood clots.

Any time a foreign object is placed in the body, there is the chance for infection. The risk is stronger with this device because it works with the blood stream.

There is a risk of clots forming in the routing hoses or the pumping mechanism. These clots can cause a heart attack, stroke or other problems. People using this device may be prescribed an anticoagulant drug such as Coumadin. However, even with the use of anticoagulant drugs, clots can still form.

Currently, LVADs are approved by the FDA for use only for people awaiting a heart transplant. Since the device must be reclassified by the FDA before it can be used on people who are not transplant recipients, its use by others is considered "experimental" and therefore, it is not widely available.

However, it is possible to be fitted with one with a little persistence, the right physical characteristics and a supportive physician. It is estimated that 70 to 80 percent of patients with end-stage CHF would benefit from using this device.

Again, because of its experimental nature, costs are not yet well known. At any rate, it would be less expensive than a heart transplant.

Cardiomyoplasty

Still in its early stages, this experimental procedure is hailed by some as a less expensive and risky alternative to transplant. In this operation, a muscle is harvested from the patient's back and wrapped around the heart. A pacemaker is implanted in the muscle to cause it to contract in the same manner as the heart.

This method may seem like a good alternative to a heart transplant – using the patient's own muscle avoids the rejection problems while giving the heart new contracting strength. But the laboratory results so far have been less encouraging.

In tests on lab animals, Cardiomioplasty has not yet been shown to significantly improve cardiac output. One problem appears to be lack of blood to the heart muscles, possibly due to the new muscle constricting the heart and pressing on the coronary arteries.

But the biggest challenge of this procedure seems to be adapting a muscle that is used for another task for use as a heart muscle. Heart muscle tissue is highly specialized and much more elastic than other muscles in the body. Because of this, the theoretical benefits of this procedure may not materialize in the near future, if ever.

Cardioversion

Cardioversion is not a treatment but an intervention tool used during crisis situations when the heart is experiencing a potentially lethal arrhythmia that has not responded to drug therapy.

The same defibrillator that delivers electric shocks to restart a heart is used for Cardioversion. Cardioversion employs a carefully timed jolt to correct the arrhythmia. The jolt depolarizes the heart – it cancels out the electrical charges built up in the heart, cleaning the electrical "slate" so the heart can start over again. Hopefully, with the proper rhythm.

Cardioversion is used as sparingly as possible because the procedure places a strain on the heart and there is a very real danger that the heart might not start beating again.

Bypass

Coronary bypass surgery is performed primarily on younger people who have CHF due to clogged coronary arteries but with no heart muscle damage.

While thousands of bypasses are performed each year, this common procedure is still a very serious operation. The sternum is sawed in half and the rib cage spread apart. The heart and lungs are then stopped and the oxygenation and circulation of the blood is performed by a heart-lung machine. A vein is harvested from the leg, attached to the aorta and grafted onto the effected coronary artery or arteries.

Between 2 and 10 percent of patients die from the operation. The death rate depends on the condition of the patient and, to a degree, the competency of the surgeons.

A bypass is an incredibly complex operation and there are many things that can go wrong. Because the entire blood supply flows through it, the heart-lung machine can be the source of many problems.

Blood clots can form while passing through the heart-lung machine and go on to cause a stroke or heart attack. About 20 percent of bypass patients suffer significant personality changes, which many think may be caused by air bubbles in the heart-lung machine that migrate to the brain.

In the best cases, the road to recovery can be a long one. It can take six months or longer to recover. Some patients never fully recover.

After a period of five years or so, the bypass can collapse, necessitating another bypass operation. These "re-ops," as they are called, are much riskier than the first operation due to the scarring of the heart from the first graft.

Having a bypass does not mean someone will not develop CHF. CHF may be caused by damage that occurred to the heart before the bypass or it may be caused by the failure of the bypass itself.

Angioplasty

The only time an angioplasty is used on someone with CHF is when they have no significant heart muscle damage and it is determined that their CHF is caused by an inadequate supply of blood to the heart muscles due to blocked arteries.

The advantages of Angioplasty over bypass operations is the reduced risk and expense of the operation when compared to a bypass. An angioplasty costs anywhere from $7,500 to $15,000, while a bypass can run from $35,000 on up, depending on complications.

In an Angioplasty, a catheter tipped with a balloon is inserted into an artery in the groin and threaded to the blocked artery in the heart. The balloon is then inflated. It pushes the blockage against the sides of the artery, widening the opening. It is then removed. The operation is performed without stopping the heart, so there is no need for a heart-lung machine.

While there is much less risk during an angioplasty operation, the procedure is not as successful as a bypass. Over a third of all arteries treated with an angioplasty collapse in the months following the operation, leaving the person as just as bad or even worse off than they were before the operation. The next step is usually a bypass operation.

Angioplasty is strongly discouraged for diabetics. Diabetes tends to cause arteries to weaken and when the artery is subjected to the stretching action of the angioplasty balloon, it simply collapses.

In fact, a recent study comparing the efficacy of bypass operations versus angioplasties in patients with diabetes was abandoned when angioplasty recipients were found to have twice the mortality rate of bypass patients.

Aneurysm

One of the top ten killers of American men over 55, aneurysms don't receive the tremendous attention that more "flashy" causes of death do.

Aneurysms are caused by atherosclerosis, the formation of plaque in the arteries. The formation of this hard plaque damages the arterial wall. The pressure of the blood coursing through the body can push on the weakened area, causing a bulge. This process can be greatly accelerated by high blood pressure, as there is more force pushing on the arterial wall.

The farther out the arterial wall bulges the weaker it becomes and, just like a balloon, the easier it can rupture. When an aneurysm ruptures, the blood flows out into the tissues, starving the area beyond the rupture of blood. This can cause shock and death in a relatively short time if it is not caught and treated.

Aneurysms can occur where the main artery branches off from the heart, called a thoracic aneurysm; or where the aorta extends down through the abdomen, called an abdominal aortic aneurysm. It can be anything from a very slight bulge to over twice the diameter of the normal artery.

How is it diagnosed?

Aneurysms are usually asymptomatic – there is no indication that the person has one or not. Two minor and seemingly unrelated symptoms that can be caused by an aneurysm are hoarseness, possibly accompanied by a dry cough, and pain in the lower back. Both of these symptoms are easily attributed to other causes and that is why most aneurysms catch the victim by surprise.

Aneurysms can be found by a variety of imaging techniques such as X-ray, Computerized Tomography (CT) scan, Magnetic Resonance Imaging (MRI), Ultrasound and many others. The problem with an aneurysm is not the difficulty of finding it, but the difficulty of knowing when to look. Many aneurysms are found while looking for other health problems.

Those who have a history of circulatory problems, such

as strokes, heart attacks and high blood pressure, should have a search for aneurysms included in their physicals and be alert for these symptoms. It is inexpensive insurance against a silent and sudden killer.

How is it treated?

Treatment depends on the location and size of the aneurysm. There are two basic options: an operation to replace the area with Dacron tubing, or the lowering of blood pressure through blood pressure drugs. The operation is a difficult and risky procedure.

An operation is indicated for abdominal aneurysms when the aneurysm measures over 2½ inches (6 centimeters) in diameter, because the possibility of death from rupture is high. There is a 50 percent chance it will burst in the next year, 75 percent within two years and 90 percent within five years.

Abdominal aneurysms less than 2 inches are treated with blood pressure drugs because they aren't as prone to rupture.

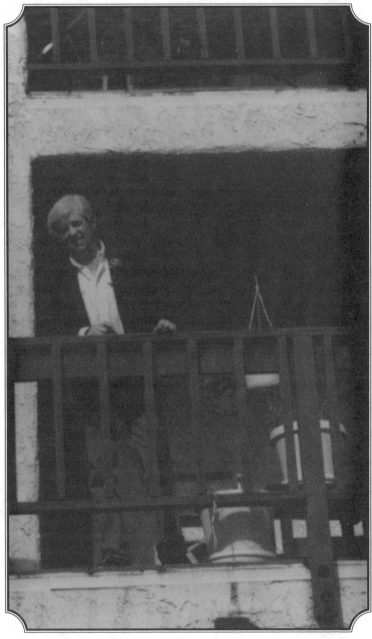

Surrounded by his herbs, Dick calls out a greeting from the balcony of his San Clemente apartment.

MEDICINES OF THE MEADOW

The art of medicine consists of amusing the patient while nature cures the disease.

-VOLTAIRE

Herbal medicine offers a wealth of ancient treatments for the modern scourge of congestive heart failure (CHF). These "green medicines" have been used to strengthen the weakened hearts of soldiers on the battlefields of the Roman Army, workers in the dank alleys of merry old England and grandmothers in the backwoods of rural America.

Herbalists wield their time-tested methods to heal the whole person, going beyond symptomatic relief to the real reason for the heart's demise. This section focuses on the use of herbal medicine for the prevention and treatment of congestive heart failure. The herbs discussed target the causes that trigger the condition while building overall cardiovascular health.

Congestive heart failure is a condition that develops over time, weakening the heart so that it can't keep up with the demands of the body for blood. As the condition progresses, blood pressure rises, the heart enlarges, fluid builds up from the ankles to the chest cavity and heart rhythm may become erratic. The causes of CHF range from chronic high blood pressure to past heart attack.

Using the herbs in this section, we hope to help those at risk avoid developing congestive heart failure by strengthening the heart and circulatory system, regulating blood pressure, clearing clogged arteries, stimulating blood flow and healing damage done by a past heart attack.

For those who already have the condition, the herbs in this chapter can strengthen the weakened heart while reducing strain; increase blood flow to starved muscles, tissues and organs; boost mental acuity while dispelling insomnia; and ease symptoms ranging from indigestion to edema (fluid retention).

The level of recovery that can be achieved using herbs depends on the condition's severity and its cause. Successful treatment requires a commitment to herbal medicine but not to the exclusion of allopathic (drug-based) medicine. Diet and lifestyle will also play an important role in supporting the herbs as they work to help the body heal itself.

HERBS AND WESTERN MEDICINE

Plants have played a major healing role in all systems of medicine for more than a millennium. Herbal treatments are employed around the world from remote villages to hi-tech science labs. Western allopathic medicine depends on chemicals found in herbs to produce most of the modern drugs on the market today.

While allopathic and herbal medicine share a few common components and can, in the case of severe congestive heart failure, complement each other for more effective treatment, there are several major differences in their approach to healing.

American medicine is trauma medicine. It is the best system in the world in emergency situations where the skills of the surgeon and the power of prescription drugs can pull the patient back from the brink of death. However, big bang drugs and invasive tests can pose more of a hazard than a benefit in the prevention or early treatment of disease.

By extracting separate chemical constituents from the herb, pharmaceuticals leave behind the plant's natural buffering agents and a host of nutrients. That's why drugs have unpleasant side-effects not found in the use of whole herbs.

Drugs prescribed to treat one condition can often cause another to develop. For example, my father was prescribed Quinidine to treat the arrhythmia (erratic heartbeat) that resulted from his severe congestive heart failure. The Physicians Desk Reference confirmed that Quinidine can cause lupus, a disease in which the immune system produces excess antibodies that attack healthy tissue.

As an herbal alternative, Hawthorn berries and Valerian root have been used for centuries to effectively treat arrhythmia – without side effects.

Designed primarily to relieve the symptoms rather than treat the cause of the condition, drugs can mask the dangerous progression of the illness by muffling the warning signals.

Drugs impose their effects artificially rather than working with the natural systems of the body. Over time, they can weaken the body's own defenses. For example, prescription diuretics drain minerals as well as excess water, resulting in potentially dangerous chemical imbalances.

"Western allopathic medicine is overkill," said herbalist James Green, author of The Male Herbal. "It bombs the body with medicine and the body has to retaliate."

Herbal medicines work from the inside out, using the body's own defense mechanisms. By tapping into the body's ability to heal itself, herbs strengthen, tone, nourish and protect without unpleasant side-effects.

For example, Dandelion is a natural diuretic that replaces lost potassium, maintaining the delicate electrolyte balance critical to proper heart rhythm. Instead of side effects, Dandelion brings the added benefit of being a blood purifier. A nutritious plant, it's high in a variety of vitamins and minerals for the heart.

Unlike drugs, most herbs do not offer a quick fix. They work gradually with a gentle healing action that leaves behind a healthier body with a renewed ability to fight disease and disability.

Mild herbal medicines such as Hawthorn are taken over a longer period of time to build lasting strength and heal the body at the deepest level. The patient must be willing to take the herbs consistently for the duration of their illness and beyond. Using herbs for prevention of congestive heart failure means making them a part of your life.

One key similarity in the philosophies of allopathic and herbal medicine is the emphasis on diet and lifestyle to maintain health and prevent disease.

Herbal medicine goes to the root of the problem but it cannot prevent recurrence of the condition if the patient reverts back to poor dietary habits or a high-stress lifestyle after completing treatment. Both allopathic doctors and herbalists recommend a well-balanced diet (see diet section), exercise and stress management to maintain good health.

In some cases, herbs can be used to wean people off harsher drug treatments for conditions such as high blood pressure, arrhythmias, edema and insomnia by solving the problem the drugs are prescribed to treat. Regular check-ups can also catch heart failure before symptoms appear or uncover "silent" causes such as elevated blood pressure for early herbal treatment.

Free of side effects, herbs can be taken alongside regular medication to help the body heal itself. Drugs become unnecessary if blood pressure stays low, heart rhythm remains regular and excess fluid does not build up.

It is important to inform your doctor of your herbal treatments so he can monitor such changes as lowered blood pressure, decreased edema and increased effectiveness of Digitalis and alter his prescriptions accordingly.

Due to the serious nature of congestive heart failure, people with the condition need to take an extremely cautious approach and seek the advice of a medical practioner before making any changes in medication.

HERBAL ALTERNATIVES TO DIGITALIS

When congestive heart failure is severe, herbs can enhance the effectiveness of the drugs but rarely replace them. The two systems of medicine can work together to increase the duration and the quality of the patient's life.

For example, Hawthorn will nourish the circulatory system and strengthen the heart muscle while maximizing the effectiveness of Digitalis. Derived from the poisonous herb Foxglove, Digitalis is a cumulative drug that builds up to a toxic level in the body over time. By taking Hawthorn, less Digitalis is needed so the dangerous accumulation is slowed.

In end-stage CHF, there are few herbs strong enough to replace Digitalis. Lily of the Valley, long considered a safer and effective herbal alternative to the highly toxic drug, is legal to use but not readily available. Concern over the herb's possible toxicity banished it from American use for so long that many people simply learned to disregard it, according to Roy Upton, president of the American Herbalists Guild.

"It's not commonly found in this market because it's considered one of the more toxic herbs but only because people forgot how to use it," Upton said. "In England, herbalists routinely use it with no problem at all. It can be used safely, but it just got lost in the cracks."

Upton, who is currently working on detailing the history and use of herbs in *The American Herbal Pharmacopoeia*, was skeptical of the studies relating to the toxicity of the plant. Those studies granted the plant a temporary place on the Food and Drug Administration's since debunked "List of 27 herbs not to use."

The dangers, Upton said, were exaggerated by experiments in which rats were fed massive amounts of cardiac glycosides isolated from the whole herb. Lily of the Valley has since been re-approved for use and can again be found among other herbs in the Merck Index.

Milder than Lily of the Valley, Night Blooming Cereus or Cactus Grandiflorus has been used by herbalists in Europe to wean patients off Digitalis, according to Upton.

Similar in action but stronger than Hawthorn, Night Blooming Cereus (Cactus Grandiflorus) has a broader range of safety than Lily of the Valley. However, Upton advised extreme caution for anyone considering substituting either herb for Digitalis.

"If you're switching from one cardiac medicine to

another you want to be closely monitored by a professional. Getting off a powerful drug can be dangerous because your body is used to it," he said. "This is not a magic bullet. There is a potential for life and death. There can be great benefit if it's done safely."

Incidentally, Digitalis is one rare case in which a derivative is preferable to using the natural herb. By synthesizing the cardiac glycosides in the leaves of the poisonous Foxglove plant, scientists standardized the dosage, making it easier to avoid accidental overdose. It's difficult to measure proper daily dosage using the natural plant leaves which vary in size, thickness and potency.

While there is no doubt Digitalis is a boon to many with severe congestive heart failure, it's a bit like being thrown a lifesaver to keep from drowning in shark-infested waters. You're safe for the moment, but the outlook still isn't good. It would be better if you hadn't fallen in at all.

The best treatment is prevention. Combining herbal supplements with a heart healthy diet can disarm the causes that trigger congestive heart failure.

Heart Herbs Deliver Multiple Benefits

Unlike most drugs, one herb can treat a variety of different ailments. Commonly used cardiac tonic herbs such as Hawthorn, Cayenne, Garlic, Ginger, Ginkgo Biloba, Motherwort and Valerian strengthen and tone the entire circulatory system while targeting the causes of CHF.

Wide spectrum herbs can do several jobs at once. For example, daily doses of Garlic will regulate blood pressure and help forestall atherosclerosis by lowering harmful cholesterol levels. Cayenne and Garlic are synergistic when taken together – each boosts the effectiveness of the other.

Working together, the two herbs clean clogged arteries like soap and water. Garlic loosens hardened cholesterol deposits on the walls of the arteries while Cayenne stimulates circulation, washing away the accumulated plaque to prevent atherosclerosis.

Aside from being a stimulant and cardiac tonic in its own right, Cayenne is also considered a "delivery herb."

Cayenne is added to countless herbal formulas because of its ability to "deliver" the healing herbs to the affected part of the body. Ginger is also a delivery herb, targeting the digestive system while dilating peripheral blood vessels to increase blood flow to the extremities.

Herbs that do "double duty," synergize together or help carry other herbs quickly to their destinations are most important in later stage congestive heart failure because circulation and digestion are sluggish. Cayenne and Ginger get the blood flowing and the herbs where they're going while delivering a few ancillary benefits of their own.

Herbs to Fight Heart Failure

There are perhaps hundreds of herbs with some benefits for people with heart failure or its causal conditions, but this chapter will concentrate on those with maximum effectiveness or the "biggest bang for the buck."

Since everybody is different, some herbs work better for some people than others. For that reason, alternate herbs with the same healing principles are included so the tonics can be tailored to the individual.

Herbs were chosen for individual power, versatility and combined benefit. For example, the diuretics in this section rid the body of excess water while purifying the blood of toxins – taking the strain off the overworked kidneys and liver.

Dosages are be designed for the level of treatment needed. Capsules of powdered herbs and teas should be used mainly for preventive therapy while tinctures (alcohol and water concentrates) are most effective in severe cases where water intake is restricted and the necessary dose of herbs is higher than capsules can deliver without discomfort.

Preventative therapy begins with regular doses of cardiac tonic herbs that build strength while treating the causes of CHF. These herbal supplements, combined with a healthy diet, exercise, stress management, regular checkups and a positive outlook; can help ward off heart failure.

Higher doses of cardiac tonics will also form basis of treatment for persons with congestive heart failure. The cardiac tonics will build the contracting strength of the heart while easing the strain on the overworked organ. However,

the first step in herbal treatment of acute illness is to eliminate hard to digest foods from the diet so the body can concentrate on healing itself . (See diet section.)

Improvement will be only temporary unless the root of
the problem is addressed. Cardiac tonic herbs also treat the
causes of congestive heart failure to help halt the progression of the condition.

Besides an in-depth look at of each of the cardiac tonic
herbs, other herbs will be discussed to treat the symptoms
of CHF that aggravate the condition such as insomnia and
edema (fluid retention).

Excessive fluid retention raises blood pressure, inhibits
breathing, slows digestion and basically, makes the patient
feel miserable all over. Diuretics have been chosen that will
not only drain the fluid but detoxify the blood, easing the
burden on the kidneys and liver.

Unlike their harsh chemical counterparts, herbal diuretics such as Dandelion replace lost potassium to maintain
the body's electrolyte balance and help prevent dangerous
arrhythmias from developing. This is another example of
how herbs work with, not against, the natural systems of
the body.

When the work is done, herbal medicines from cardiac
tonics to diuretics leave behind nourishment while drugs
deposit toxins. Blood purifying and nourishing herbs have
been included to help the body heal itself.

Herbalists believe that the healing process generates an
increased amount of waste that builds up in the blood and
tissues. If the body is unable to rid itself of these natural
wastes, it becomes congested. This congestion blocks the
delivery of nutrients needed for healing and so, inhibits
recovery.

Blood purifiers remove wastes by boosting metabolism,
increasing circulation, stimulating kidney and liver function, opening the pores and assuring bowel regularity.

Feeding the body properly is just as important as dis-
posing of waste. Included in this section are herbs high in
essential nutrients for cardiovascular health. These herbs,
which include Kelp and Alfalfa, will help build back the
strength sapped by congestive heart failure. Tonic herbs like
Ginseng and Fo-ti will help restore vitality while sedatives
like Valerian (also a cardiac tonic), Passion Flower and Hops

deliver refreshing rest.

Since the use of drugs like Digitalis are critical for people with late-stage heart failure, many of the herbs in this section enhance or complement prescription medicines. For example, Hawthorn maximizes the effectiveness of Digitalis and Garlic is a natural vasodilator. Vasodilators reduce high blood pressure by preventing constriction of the blood vessels. Other natural vasodilators and cardiac stimulants are included in this chapter to assist in the overall treatment.

CARDIAC TONICS COMBAT HEART FAILURE

Cardiac tonic blends nourish, strengthen, tone and regulate the circulatory system from head to toe. They form the basis for good cardiac health and the first line of defense against congestive heart failure. For those with heart failure, cardiac tonics can help halt the progression of the condition and enhance their quality of life.

In Germany, physicians commonly prescribe cardiac tonics at the first sign of cardiovascular disease to avert potential problems, rather than waiting for the condition to reach a crisis and resorting to drugs or surgery as their American counterparts often do.

Taken regularly, cardiac tonics can help protect the circulatory system from damage due to muscular degeneration, clogged arteries, weakened capillary walls and free radical scavengers.

By far, the most commonly prescribed cardiac tonic herb is Hawthorn berry. While it works well when taken with other herbs in a cardiac tonic mixture, supplemental doses of this gentle herb are recommended for people who already have heart failure.

For nourishing, strengthening and regenerating the heart, nothing beats Hawthorn. It increases the power of each heart muscle contraction, normalizes heart rhythm and increases circulation by dilating both the coronary arteries and the peripheral blood vessels. Adding Cayenne will boost the power of the Hawthorn as the two herbs are synergistic.

Hawthorn combined with Linden Blossom or Garlic is

an effective treatment of atherosclerosis. Garlic, Cayenne and Hawthorn regulate blood pressure to treat both a cause and a symptom of CHF. Paired with Valerian, Hawthorn eases angina and helps regulate heart rhythm.

While Hawthorn feeds the veins and arteries to retain the elasticity of youth, Valerian and Motherwort help control the neurological functions of the heart and blood vessels. Ginger and Ginkgo Biloba help dilate the tiny capillaries, assuring peripheral blood flow for mental acuity, digestion, muscle strength and warmth in the extremities.

Stimulants like Cayenne and Ginger increase oxygenation of the muscles, tissues and organs while Hawthorn increases the heart's ability to metabolize oxygen and nutrients so it needs less to do more. Kelp contains high levels of oxygen and nutrients to nourish systems throughout the body.

Ginger stimulates the digestive system to aid assimilation of nutrients while Dandelion and other blood purifying diuretics rid the body of excess water and toxins. Cramp Bark and Valerian relax tense muscles and soothe a frayed nervous system.

Blends combining the most commonly used cardiac tonic herbs in Western herbalism: Hawthorn, Cayenne, Garlic, Ginger, Ginkgo Biloba, Motherwort and Linden Blossom are the cornerstone of the prevention and treatment of Congestive Heart Failure.

CARDIAC TONIC FORMULAS

Dr. Daniel Mowrey, herbalist and author of *The Scientific Validation of Herbal Medicine* and other works, recommends a nutritional cardiac tonic to help prevent or reduce the severity of a variety of heart conditions including congestive heart failure.

Mowrey's cardiac tonic blend mixes equal parts of Hawthorn berries, Motherwort, Rosemary leaves, Kelp and Cayenne. He recommends taking 2-4 capsules per day as a heart tonic.

For people who already have congestive heart failure, David Hoffmann, teacher, herbalist, past president of the American Herbalists Guild and author of *An Elder's Herbal*, recommends daily doses of Garlic and a cardiac tonic made up of 3 parts Hawthorn, 1 part Ginkgo Biloba, 1 part Linden Blossom, 1 part Dandelion Leaf, 1 part Motherwort and 1 part Cramp Bark.

Taken as an alcohol-based tincture to ease digestion or abide by dietary water restriction, Hoffmann suggests 1 teaspoon doses 3 times a day. To make an infusion, take 2 tablespoons of the dried herb blend and steep 10-15 minutes in a cup of hot water. Drink 3 cups a day.

Dr. John Christopher, hailed as the "Patron Saint of Cayenne Pepper," recommended the use of all these cardiac tonic herbs driven by the power of the hot red pepper.

Besides taking Cayenne and Garlic capsules four times daily, Christopher suggested an infusion made by steeping 2 ounces of Motherwort and one ounce Hawthorn in $1\frac{1}{2}$ pints of boiling water in a tightly covered container for 15 minutes. He recommends patients drink one wine glass full 3-4 times a day.

Dick Quinn's heart formula for congestive heart failure relied heavily on hard-to-get Lily of the Valley as he knew it was one of the few viable substitutes for Digitalis.

A self-taught herbalist and author of *Left For Dead*, Quinn blends 60 percent Lily of the Valley, 30 percent Hawthorn, 15 percent Rosemary and 5 percent Cayenne. He recommended up to 4,000 mg or 8 capsules per day to treat severe CHF.

Roy Upton suggested a basic cardiac tonic mixture using Night Blooming Cereus or Cactus Grandiflorus instead of the rarer Lily of the Valley. Upton's recipe for prevention is a syrup made from combining blackstrap molasses with 4 parts Hawthorn, 2-3 parts Night Blooming Cereus (Cactus Grandiflorus), 1 part Motherwort and 2-3 parts specific tonic herbs.

The final ingredient depends on the effect desired. It could be Linden Blossom to ease nervous tension and lower blood pressure, Ginseng to increase stamina or Red Clover to thin the blood.

"It's the Julia Child School of Herbalism," Upton joked of the formula's flexibility. "It's about using what you have when you're making it. You take the base formula – it's a general heart tonic – and what you add depends on the specific needs of the person taking it."

Using the cardiac tonic as a syrup creates more of a nourishing tonic than a medicine, Upton said. Blackstrap molasses nourishes the blood which passes the benefits on to the heart as it moves through. As a preventative, he suggests 1 teaspoon of the syrup twice a day, morning and evening.

For more acute cases, Upton, who practiced herbalism for seven years, employed the same mixture in tincture form. Higher in alcohol than the syrup, the tincture formula was more readily absorbed. He suggests 15-30 drops of the tincture twice a day.

Each of the herbs mentioned above will be explored in this chapter along with suggestions for individual use to supplement the cardiac tonic formulas of Mowrey, Hoffmann, Christopher, Quinn and Upton or to create your own mixture according to your individual needs.

PROCURING AND PREPARING HERBAL MEDICINES

The herbs in this chapter can be taken in a variety of ways. They can be eaten hot or cold in food, sipped in teas or tinctures, or taken in a pill, capsule or syrup.

Medicinal teas known as infusions and decoctions use water to draw the healing properties out of the herb. Tinctures use a mixture of water and alcohol to dissolve and preserve the healing oils in the herb. Capsules contain powdered whole herbs and make it easier to ingest hot or distasteful herbs.

Medicinal decoctions and infusions are much stronger than the weak herbal teas sold in grocery stores. The grocery store beverages contain only about 1/7 of an ounce of herb and will do little but please the palate. Medicinal infusions and decoctions use 1 ounce of dried herb per pint (2 cups) of water and are taken in half or full cup doses usually three times a day.

Infusions are most commonly used for more delicate plant parts such as leaves, flowers and soft stems. Since the herb is steeped rather than boiled, valuable essential oils are preserved. Harder plants like Valerian and Burdock Root are best steeped or simmered gently to preserve the volatile oils that contain their healing principals.

Just like the contents of a tea bag, dried herbs are usually used for an infusion; however fresh plants can be substituted by tripling the measure. For fresh herbs, use your hands or a mortar and pestle to bruise the leave, stem or stalk to release the active components.

To make an herbal infusion, put one teaspoon (1/2 ounce) of dried or three teaspoons of fresh herb in a warm teapot. Add one cup of boiling distilled or spring water, cover tightly and steep for 10-15 minutes. Strain, sweeten to taste and serve hot or cold. Hawthorn, Linden Blossom and Peppermint make good infusions.

In a decoction, herbs are exposed to higher heat to unlock the medicinal properties contained in hard woody bark, stems, nuts and roots. In a large glass, enamel or earthenware pot place 1 teaspoon of dried herbs or three teaspoons of fresh herbs for each cup of water. Bring mixture to a boil. Cover and simmer for up to 15 minutes, depending on the fragility of the herb. Strain while still hot.

For formulas containing both course and delicate herbs, make a decoction using the harder plants, strain and pour over softer plants to make an infusion. Steep for 10-20 minutes and strain again.

Woody herbs high in volatile oils like Valerian and Burdock Root can be powdered and made into an infusion or tincture to preserve their medicinal properties. Infusions and decoctions can be made in volume, stored in the refrigerator for up to three days and re-heated slowly in a covered pot.

In many cases, herb tinctures are preferable to infusions and decoctions because alcohol often draws out the medicinal properties of plants more effectively than water while preserving delicate volatile oils.

Stronger than their watery counterparts, drops of tincture can be taken alone, mixed in juice or added to water. They work well with a CHF patient's water-restricted diet and sluggish digestion while making bitter herbs more palatable. Tincture doses vary from a few drops to a couple teaspoons depending on the herb and the severity of the ailment.

To make a tincture, measure four ounces of dried or eight ounces fresh herbs and place in a container with a tight seal. Pour in 1 pint of Vodka, Brandy, Gin or Rum and close the lid tightly. Keep the mixture in a warm dark place for two weeks, shaking once a day. Strain the tincture through cheese cloth or a filter into a dark bottle with a tight seal.

Wine can also be used to make the tincture. Flavorful and effective, herbs infused in wine do not have as long a shelf life as tinctures with a higher alcohol content. If alcohol is completely restricted, tinctures can be made from the same recipe using vinegar. They can also be made using glycerin.

Glycerin-based tinctures are not as strong medicinally as alcohol-based tinctures but they are often easier on the digestive system. Glycerin dissolves the plant's constituents better than water but not as thoroughly as alcohol.

To make a Glycerin tincture, herbalist David Hoffmann combines a half pint each of glycerin and water and adds four ounces of dried herb. The mixture is allowed to sit in a sealed container for two weeks and shaken daily. The contents are then strained. For fresh herbs, use eight ounces of the plant in a mixture of 75 percent glycerin and 25 percent water.

Herbal extracts found in health food stores are not the same as tinctures. Instead, they use solvents to extract the major components from the herb. These extracts are up to 10 times more concentrated than ordinary tinctures and are often taken in doses of 6-8 drops to each teaspoon of tincture.

Cardiac tonics can also be taken in a nourishing syrup using blackstrap molasses to draw the healing properties from the herb. The syrup can be made by adding 2 cups of herb tea (decoction or infusion) to 3/4 pound of molasses or adding one part tincture to three parts blackstrap molasses.

Syrups using blackstrap molasses as a base can contain as much as 20 percent alcohol. Taking herbs in a syrup can sweeten bitter concoctions and add nutrients from the blackstrap molasses. As a preventative, the usual syrup dosage is 1 teaspoon a day.

Capsules and tablets have made it possible to take larger quantities of whole herbs regardless of taste or texture. The drawback is that rapid and complete absorption is not guaranteed.

Heat, water and alcohol are used to pull out the healing properties of the herb in infusions, decoctions and tinctures. The digestive juices may not break down the herbal constituents as well or as quickly. In a liquid form, herbs may be more readily absorbed and act faster than powdered plants taken as a capsule or tablet. This makes the addition of catalyst and carrier herbs important in dried blends.

Since capsules contain only about 1/6 of an ounce of herbs, they should be used for more powerful herbs such as Cayenne pepper and Garlic. A typical dose is two capsules three times a day.

Milder herbs such as Hawthorn can be added to blends with catalyst herbs like Cayenne but may be more effective in tinctures and infusions when heart failure is acute and larger doses are necessary. Large doses of powdered herbs taken in gelatin capsules can lead to indigestion and aggravate an already sluggish digestive system.

A wide range of pre-packaged herbal combinations are available in health and drug stores. However, if you'd like to make your own capsules or produce your own teas and tinctures, you can purchase herbs and "00" size gelatin capsules in health stores, co-ops and certain specialty grocery stores.

Whether you take herbs in capsules, teas or tincture, what's most important is that you take them. Herbs like Hawthorn impart their benefits over time and must be taken in sufficient doses to safeguard cardiovascular health. On the other hand, Cayenne's effects are felt immediately, but are not as long-lasting.

The next section will explain the medicinal uses of each herb and how it relates to an herbal program for the prevention and treatment of congestive heart failure.

Herbs for the Heart

Cardiac Tonic Stimulants

Hawthorn (Latin name: *Crataegus Oxyacantha*)

This heart tonic can be eaten on toast. A popular marmalade in Europe, Hawthorn increases the heart's pumping action, strengthens the heart muscle, lowers high blood pressure, eases angina, speeds recovery from heart attack and strengthens the entire circulatory system.

Native to the Mediterranean, North America, Europe

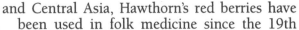

and Central Asia, Hawthorn's red berries have been used in folk medicine since the 19th century for the treatment of congestive heart failure and the causes of the condition including high blood pressure, atherosclerosis, irregular heart beat and inflammation of the heart muscle.

As a preventative, Hawthorn guards against cardiovascular degeneration by toning the heart muscle and strengthening the arteries, veins and capillaries. Hawthorn can help prevent heart disease from developing and restore the elasticity of youth to the circulatory system.

An intensive four-year study by the German Federal Ministry of Health hailed Hawthorn as a remedy for a variety of heart problems. The Ministry study concluded the herb was especially effective in treating "loss of cardiac function," congestion and "oppression" of the heart and arrhythmias.

The healing properties found in the leaves, root, flowers and fruit also lower cholesterol, de-acidify the blood, act as a mild diuretic, relieve insomnia and aid digestion.

A double-blind study performed in 1981 on patients with heart failure documented Hawthorn's ability to boost heart function. However, therapeutic benefits are contained in the whole plant. Isolated constituents have proven ineffective.

Experiments conducted in several countries, including the United States, Germany and Hungary, show Hawthorn acts as a natural vasodilator. Flavonoids in the herb dilate the coronary arteries and the blood vessels away from the heart, lowering peripheral resistance to blood flow and thereby regulating blood pressure.

Hawthorn's ability to regulate heart beat and control arrhythmias was documented in the acclaimed monographs (therapeutic guidelines) of the German Commission E published in 1983.

One study showed intravenous injections of Hawthorn extract reduced tachycardia (rapid heartbeat) within 20 minutes, according to herbalist Rudolph Weiss, author of *Herbal Medicine*. In less acute cases, oral doses of

Hawthorn proved effective with either tachycardia or bradycardia (slow heartbeat), Weiss wrote.

Hawthorn also enhances the flexibility of veins and arteries which helps keep blood pressure down. Increased blood flow to the heart itself reduces the incidence of angina.

Besides easing the burden congestive heart failure places on the heart, Hawthorn boosts the heart's ability to metabolize oxygen, nutrients and enzymes in the blood. In a study of 50 heart patients on a mild exercise regime, those taking the herb were able to reduce their oxygen consumption 77 percent compared to 25 percent for those using standard treatments.

Increasing the efficiency of oxygen consumption, Hawthorn strengthens and tones the heart muscle itself enhancing the power of each contraction. In essence, the heart is able to pump more blood with less effort.

While providing more nourishment to perform the job at hand, Hawthorn also stabilizes rhythm to keep the heart from working against itself. It has been used effectively to treat tachycardia and other arrythmias that arise in congestive heart failure.

Recently, experiments have debunked the long-held belief that Hawthorn's effect on the heart duplicates the drug Digitalis which is made from the herb Foxglove. The chemical constituents of the two herbs are different. Hawthorn does not contain cardiac-glycosides, the active ingredient in Digitalis.

There are several critical differences in the way Hawthorn and Digitalis work. Hawthorn lowers blood pressure by dilating peripheral blood vessels while Digitalis acts directly on the heart. In patients with severe congestive heart failure, Hawthorn's effects are not immediately felt, unlike Digitalis.

However, studies show the herb regulates the heart's action and increases cardiac output over time without accumulating in the system like Digitalis. Unlike Hawthorn, Digitalis is toxic and must be closely monitored to avoid a deadly overdose.

Taken together, Hawthorn and Digitalis enhance each other's potency. Researchers found treating heart tissue with one of the substances greatly increased the effectiveness of the other. Only half the normal dosage was required for full effect when the two were combined.

Digitalis works on the symptoms of congestive heart failure, not the cause. It stimulates the weakened heart muscle to increase the power of each contraction without any lasting health benefits to the heart itself. It does not heal or protect the damaged heart, as Hawthorn does. Hawthorn assists Digitalis by providing more nourishment and oxygen to the stimulated muscle. In the same way, Hawthorn has also proven to augment the effects of Strophanthin, a German heart medication derived from an African herb.

Germany's Commission E also cited Hawthorn's success in the treatment of stage one and stage two congestive heart failure. By increasing coronary circulation while stabilizing heart rhythm, the nourishing cardiac tonic herb greatly benefited elderly patients who had not yet gotten to the point where Digitalis was necessary, Commission E reported.

Called "the cure for the aging heart" Hawthorn must be taken in sufficient doses over a long period of time to properly safeguard the circulatory system or act as an effective therapy in the treatment of congestive heart failure. This gentle healing herb is not meant to be used for short-term treatment or emergency intervention. It can take weeks for the patient to feel the difference. While the results are not rapid, the benefits are long-lasting.

Whether Hawthorn is taken as a tincture, infusion or capsule, it's important the preparation contain the whole herb as studies have shown the isolated constituents are ineffective.

Hawthorn is nontoxic, non-addictive, not cumulative and remarkably free of side effects. However, in rare cases, high doses of Hawthorn can cause dizziness and nausea. This can be remedied by taking the herb during or immediately following meals.

To treat acute CHF, an infusion can made from 2 teaspoons of the dried herb per cup of water and taken three times a day. If using a tincture, herbalist David Hoffmann suggests 30-40 drops three times daily to see immediate results and up to 100 drops twice a day for up to six weeks for acute conditions. A therapeutic tincture dose would be 30-40 drops in the morning and evening, Hoffmann wrote.

Hawthorn is the main ingredient in Hoffmann's cardiac tonic for congestive heart failure. The herbalist and author blends 3 parts Hawthorn with one part each of Ginkgo Biloba, Linden Blossom, Dandelion leaf, Motherwort and Cramp Bark. Taken as a tincture, he suggests 1 teaspoon three times a day. As an infusion, use 2 teaspoons per cup of hot water and drink three cups a day.

Dr. John Christopher recommends a heart tonic made from 1 ounce Hawthorn berry and 2 ounces Motherwort. Infuse the herbs in 1½ pints boiling water for 15 minutes then strain. Drink 1 wineglass full 3-4 times a day.

Motherwort (Latin name: *Leonurus Cardiaca*)

Called "the heart herb," Motherwort strengthens heart function while calming palpitations, improves circulation and boosts overall cardiac health. It also regulates blood pressure, eases diarrhea and quells depression.

Since the herb's Latin name "Cardiaca" is taken from the Greek word for heart, it's not surprising that Motherwort was employed by ancient Greeks and Romans to treat both the emotional and the physical ailments of the heart ranging from palpitations to depression.

English herbalist John Gerard wrote of the herb as a remedy for "infirmities of the heart" in the 16th century. Gerard's 17th century counterpart, herbalist Nicholas Culpepper, recommended it for "tremblings of the heart."

While their Western neighbors were using the stems, flowers and leaves to "strengthen and gladden the heart," Chinese practitioners were touting the plant as a longevity herb.

According to an ancient Chinese legend, a boy was banished to a remote valley where Motherwort grew in profusion alongside a spring. He is said to have lived to the ripe old age of 300.

Ancient claims that Motherwort calms palpitations was borne out recently by test tube studies in China showing that the herb relaxes heart cells. Additional study showed the herb may also inhibit the formation of heart attack-causing blood clots.

The herb's high calcium content may account for its

effectiveness in treating arrhythmia since the mineral helps regulate the rhythm of the heart beat. Preliminary findings by Russian researchers show Motherwort contains glycosides which lower blood pressure. Tannins in the herb stop diarrhea.

Like other tonics, Motherwort has soothing sedative and antispasmodic properties. While calming the heart and the nervous system, Motherwort also strengthens a weakened heart. It has been used to treat inflammations of the heart muscle (endocarditis and pericarditis) and as a diuretic, it can reduce the burden edema places on the heart, liver and kidneys.

Gentle on the system, Motherwort can be taken safely in high doses over a long period of time – much like Hawthorn.

An infusion of 1-2 teaspoons of the dried herb steeped for 10 minutes can be taken two or three times a day. Sweeten to taste with sugar, lemon or honey as Motherwort has a bitter flavor. A tincture dosage of 1/2 to 1 teaspoon can be taken 3 times a day.

Mowrey's cardiac tonic blends equal parts of Motherwort, Hawthorn berry, Rosemary leaf, Kelp and Cayenne. He suggests 2-4 capsules be taken per day to help prevent heart disease-related conditions like CHF or reduce the severity of the symptoms.

Cayenne Pepper (Latin name: *Capsicum annum*)

Searching for a new spice route, explorer Christopher Columbus discovered the bright red fruit that bites back. On his second voyage, he was accompanied by a physician who chronicled the many medicinal uses of the potent spice. Since then, Cayenne or Capsicum has been regaled as the perfect stimulant for the entire body.

Targeting the heart first, Cayenne spreads its benefits to the rest of the body through the arteries, capillaries and nerves. High blood pressure drops as the herb clears clogged veins, regulating blood flow from head to toe.

Nourishing the veins, arteries and capillaries, Cayenne restores elasticity so each heartbeat pulses with more power. For those with congestive heart failure,

Cayenne stimulates the weakened heart without straining the overburdened organ.

Cayenne invigorates the heart, increases circulation, boosts the power of each heartbeat, regulates blood pressure and helps the circulatory system regain its youthful flexibility by feeding the cell structure of the arteries, veins and capillaries.

In a dramatic impromptu demonstration, Dr. John Christopher showed how the powerful pepper can stop even a heart attack in progress by putting a mixture of Cayenne and water under the tongue of a man stricken during one of the herbalist's seminars. According to the story, the man was back on his feet before the ambulance arrived.

As a catalyst herb, Cayenne enhances the effectiveness of other herbs. It speeds delivery and aids absorption by stimulating the circulatory and digestive systems.

Used in a plethora of herbal products ranging from laxatives to cough medicine, a little bit of Cayenne helps other herbs go a long way toward healing. Added to Ginger, Cayenne helps clean out the bronchial tubes. For respiratory infections, combining Cayenne and Garlic speeds up the antibiotic action of the other herb so much that it's akin to taking liquid penicillin.

Working together, Cayenne and Garlic act like soap and water to cleanse the circulatory system and clear blocked arteries. Studies show Garlic oil penetrates hardened deposits, loosening them so they can be washed away by the soapy vitamin A in Cayenne. This type of circulatory housekeeping is important since blocked arteries and the resulting high blood pressure are two primary causes of congestive heart failure.

In an ordinary diet, Cayenne can prevent the absorption of cholesterol. In an experiment conducted at the Central Food Technological Research Institute of Mysore, India, two groups of rats were fed a high cholesterol diet. The test group that was given Cayenne showed no rise in liver cholesterol levels and in fact, excreted the cholesterol.

Protein appears critical to Cayenne's ability to fight cholesterol. Researchers found the herb was unable to reduce cholesterol levels significantly for people eating a low protein/high fat diet. However, Cayenne inhibited cholesterol absorption for patients eating a higher amount of protein.

Possessing the same chemical found in other cholesterol-blocking plants such as Alfalfa, Garlic and Ginger, Cayenne appears to deactivate bile salts necessary to absorb cholesterol through the intestinal wall.

Dispelling artery-clogging cholesterol is only one way Cayenne keeps the circulatory system free of obstructions that could trigger heart attack or stroke and precipitate congestive heart failure.

A chemical called fibrin causes the blood to clot. A certain amount of the chemical is necessary to ensure small wounds are not fatal, but too much fibrin can cause deadly clots to form. The process of ridding the body of excess fibrin is called fibrinosis. Studies have shown Cayenne stimulates fibrinosis and reduces the chance of clot-caused heart attack or stroke.

In countries where Capsicum is a regular part of the diet such as Thailand, India, Korea and East Africa, the incidence of heart disease is strikingly low.

High in the mountains of Asia Minor, the Hunzas tribe live on a diet centered around mineral-rich water, apricots and fresh Cayenne Peppers. With this hot and sour menu, the Hunzas live to be over 100 years old and can be seen playing polo at age 150. The major cause of death is from a fall rather than the ravages of disease.

The redder the pepper, the more vitamin A (beta carotene) it contains. Paprika, the mildest Capsicum, has the highest vitamin C content. Drying Cayenne depletes the herb of vitamin C so the highest amount of that heart healthy antioxidant can be found in fresh peppers.

Minerals in the fruit, including calcium, magnesium, phosphorus, sulfur and iron; help make it an effective treatment for heart disease, arthritis, pancreatic and throat disorders.

As a cardiac tonic, Cayenne strengthens and protects the entire circulatory system, regulates blood pressure and boosts the power of the heart by easing the flow of blood throughout the body.

By cleansing the circulatory system, the powerful pepper increases blood flow to the digestive and respiratory systems, the nerves and the brain. By stimulating the flow of gastric juices, saliva, urine and perspiration, Cayenne helps the body assimilate nutrients and rid itself of wastes. All functions of the body are improved by Cayenne from digestion to eyesight.

For those at risk of heart failure, Cayenne can help strengthen the circulatory system while targeting CHF causes such as atherosclerosis and high blood pressure. Patients who already have CHF can benefit from increased energy, better digestion, enhanced circulation and a more forceful heartbeat.

It's important to note that whole herb Cayenne is greater than the sum of its parts. In 1876 scientists isolated Capsaicin, the central chemical in Cayenne. Extracts of Capsaicin do not duplicate the action of the whole herb and in fact, can do just the opposite. The whole herb contains natural buffering agents that are lost when one ingredient is extracted.

For example, Cayenne has been shown to lower high blood pressure, but Capsaicin can boost it. Capsaicin can cause hypertension, slow the heart rate and damage cells in the gastrointestinal system preventing absorption of nutrients from food.

Beneficial Capsicum can be found in the hottest to mildest chili peppers and even cool paprika. The potency of pepper is measured in heat units. The hottest Cayenne is found in Sierra Leone. African Birdseye Cayenne is rated at up to 150,000 heat units while Tabasco sauce is about 25,000 heat units and cooking Cayenne comes in at 2,000 heat units.

With the advent of the gelatin capsule, even those who cannot eat spicy food can take the hottest Cayenne. However, the heat of the pepper was a natural deterrent to overindulgence. Pepper novices should build a tolerance slowly and add Ginger to put out the fire. Remember, Cayenne works best when combined with a diet low in fat and high in protein and complex carbohydrates.

In addition to capsules, Cayenne can be eaten in food, sipped in a tea, rubbed in as an ointment or packed in a poultice. Cayenne mixed with oil and rubbed into the soles of the feet has been shown to restore circulation in diabetics.

Cayenne can be stored for up to a year in a sealed wax or plastic container at room temperature. Paper bags will leech out the precious oil. Also, decoctions will boil away Cayenne's essential oils and the medicinal properties will be lost. Instead, make an infusion by pouring a cup of hot water over 1 teaspoon of the pepper.

Dr. John Christopher recommends starting with small doses of the infusion and increasing gradually to allow the body to become acclimated to the powerful pepper.

Christopher's regimen begins with 1/4 teaspoon of the infusion three times a day. On the third day increase the dose to 1/2 teaspoon three times a day. Add 1/4 teaspoon when palatable to reach the minimum recommended daily dose of one full teaspoon three times per day.

Cayenne should be taken in capsules, alone or with other herbs, at least twice per day as a maintenance dose to help prevent CHF. For those with heart failure, two capsules of Cayenne heart tonic blends are recommended three times a day.

Combining Cayenne with Hawthorn produces a synergism that boosts the effectiveness of both cardiac tonic herbs. For example, while Hawthorn is the "heart" of Mowrey's cardiac tonic blend, Cayenne is the delivery vehicle that speeds it to the ailing organ.

Adding Garlic lowers blood pressure and clears clogged arteries. Mild cardiac tonic herbs like Motherwort and Rosemary derive extra power when mixed with Cayenne.

Garlic (Latin name: *Allium Sativum*)

This pungent member of the Lily family has been used since ancient times to treat ailments of the circulatory system, including congestive heart failure and its causes.

Hippocrates was using Garlic to treat angina in 460 B.C. Dioscorides, physician to the Roman armies in the first century A.D., listed Garlic as a treatment for edema. At the same time, physicians in India were using it to ward off heart disease and rheumatism.

Garlic regulates circulation by lowering high blood pressure and raising low blood pressure. It is also used to strengthen the heart, quell heart palpitations and expand blood vessel walls. It boosts energy, acts as a natural antibiotic and stimulates the digestive tract. It reduces harmful cholesterol and loosens fatty deposits that collect in the arteries.

Regular ingestion of Garlic may reduce the chance of contracting congestive heart failure by alleviating atherosclerosis and high blood pressure.

Numerous experiments performed in universities and hospitals from Japan to Germany have proven Garlic lowers harmful cholesterol levels. Herbalists, chemists and physicians all tout Garlic's value in the fight against heart disease.

Ten years ago, the results of a study were published comparing three groups of vegetarians on similar diets in India who ate large amounts, small amounts and no amounts of Garlic and Onion over a long period of time. The levels of serum cholesterol were lowest in those who ate the most Garlic/Onion and highest in those who ate none at all. Abstainers' blood also clotted more quickly.

Another study compared two groups of patients with coronary artery disease over a 10-month period. The levels of low density lipoproteins – a sign of heart disease – steadily declined in the group taking Garlic supplements. Garlic lowers blood pressure, sugars, lipids, free cholesterol and low density lipoproteins while raising beneficial high density lipoproteins.

Garlic also reduces the chances of heart attack and stroke by inhibiting the ability of blood cells to stick together to form clots. One experiment took a group of vegetarians that were of the same age, sex, and social class and separated them according to whether or not they ate Garlic.

The cholesterol levels of both groups were low since they did not eat meat, but the group that ate Garlic also had less clot-causing fibrinogen and other substances that trigger atherosclerosis such as serum triglycerides.

Garlic may protect the heart from damage caused by drugs and alcohol – another cause of congestive heart failure. Researchers injected two groups of rats with isoproterenol, a drug known to cause heart damage. Autopsies performed on the rats who were given Garlic in their diet showed dramatically fewer lesions on their heart muscles than those who had not consumed Garlic.

The odorous herb is rich in nutrients – high in vitamins A and C, protein, thiamin and numerous trace minerals including potassium, calcium, selenium, zinc and iron. Its volatile oils make it a natural vasodilator, holding blood vessels open wide to keep blood pressure down.

Garlic is one of the most effective herbal agents for lowering high blood pressure. More importantly, it can treat the cause of high blood pressure itself by expanding the blood vessel walls and nurturing the health of the blood vessels themselves.

People who have high blood pressure or atherosclerosis or just have the genetic disposition to develop it should make Garlic a part of their daily life in the hope of averting these conditions and ultimately, avoiding congestive heart failure.

Garlic can be eaten in food, sipped in tea or juice, ingested in capsule form but should never be boiled as that destroys the active components of the herb. Raw Garlic kills bacteria and boosts the immune system. Cooked garlic lowers cholesterol, thins the blood and acts as an expectorant and decongestant.

The fresher the herb and more pungent the aroma, the stronger the effect as Garlic's medicinal value comes from the chemical reaction that raises the stink. When the bulb is cut or bruised, the enzyme alliinase mixes with alliin to form allicin. Garlic's curative powers come from allicin.

In Italy, where Garlic is a culinary cornerstone, sprigs of Parsley are eaten as breath fresheners. While chlorophyll in the herb absorbs the odor in Garlic, Parsley is also a recommended herb for congestive heart failure. It is a nutritious diuretic often prescribed by herbalists as a tonic for the blood vessels because it is high in vitamins A and B. Gentle as it is effective, Parsley soothes irritations of the liver, kidney and spleen.

Cooked or raw, in drops or capsules, it's not as important how you take Garlic as that you take it.

Since Garlic and Cayenne synergize to boost each other's effectiveness, it's a good idea to take a blend that includes both if you are taking Garlic in capsule form.

Hoffmann suggests Garlic be taken to supplement his cardiac tonic for congestive heart failure. As a preventative, he suggests 4 grams – about a clove per day. For those who do not like fresh Garlic, supplements are available that contain at least 10 milligrams of allicin or a total allicin potential of 4,000 micrograms that are as effective as the fresh herb.

Mowrey recommends high blood pressure capsules made up of Garlic, Cayenne, Valerian Root, Black Cohosh Root (an herbal vasodilator) and Kelp to reduce high blood pressure, lower cholesterol and relieve nervous anxiety.

He suggests taking 2-3 capsules of his blood pressure blend three to four times per day to treat acute conditions.

As a preventative, he recommends 1-2 blood pressure capsules be taken to supplement 2-4 capsules of his heart blend, described in the cardiac tonics section.

Onion (Latin name: *Allium Cepa*)

Medicinally similar to Garlic, Onion has been touted for centuries as a heart tonic, blood thinner, blood purifier, diuretic and digestive aid.

Onions reduce the risk of heart attack and stroke by regulating cholesterol levels. Studies performed by Dr. Victor Gurewich, a leading cardiologist and a professor at Tufts University in Boston, showed that the juice of a single white or yellow Onion taken daily raised HDL cholesterol by at least 30 percent.

HDL (high density lipoprotein) cholesterol is the "good cholesterol" that protects against heart disease by removing dangerous excess LDL (low density lipoprotein) cholesterol from the blood and sending it to the liver where it can be destroyed. Low HDL levels increase the risk of heart attack. Gurewich found that the fresher the raw Onion, the more dramatic the increase, but that cooked onions had little effect on cholesterol levels.

Cooked or raw onions both contain adenosine, a compound that inhibits the tendency of platelets to stick together and form clots. Onion also stimulates the fibrinolyic system to dissolve blood clots that have already formed. The blood thinning properties of Onions have been long known by the French who added them to their horse's diet to break up clots in the legs.

A tablespoon of cooked Onions or two ounces raw will help mitigate the damage caused by a high fat meal, according to a 1966 study performed at the K.G. Medical College in Lucknow, India.

Foods high in saturated fat have been shown to increase clot-forming fibrinogen, thicken the blood and boost the level of bad LDL cholesterol. Just two ounces of Onion added to a meal packed with butter, cream and eggs counteracts these effects by stimulating the fibrinolyic system and the HDL cholesterol level to help rid the body of these fat-induced dangers.

A 1923 study showed that Onion also lowers blood

sugar. Whether raw, cooked or in extract form, Indian researchers found Onion lowered blood sugar in patients who had just taken glucose. Regulating blood sugar is critical to cardiac health. (See Diet section.)

A nutritious part of a balanced diet, Onions are high in heart healthy magnesium, potassium, protein and anticarcinogen vitamins A and C.

For his heart patients, Dr. Gurewich prescribed an Onion a day to keep the doctor away. As with Garlic, the general rule is "the more the better." Onion benefits those best who eat it most. Cooked or raw, a cup of onions a day will keep the circulatory system in good shape and offer a defense against congestive heart failure.

Ginger (Latin name: *Zingiber Officinale*)

A mild stimulant, Ginger moves back and forth from the capillaries through the veins to the heart producing a feeling of warmth. More diffuse than Cayenne, Ginger reaches the peripheral areas and concentrates on the digestive organs.

Like Cayenne, it is a good delivery herb. Adding Ginger to formulas speeds other herbs to their targeted areas – especially the digestive system.

As a tonic, Ginger stimulates the circulatory system, cleanses the blood, aids digestion and eases motion and morning sickness.

Ginger is a good preventative herb for heart failure and its many causes. Those who already have the condition will benefit from increased peripheral circulation and better digestion. Detoxifying the blood will help safeguard the health of the heart muscle tissues.

Studies performed in the former Soviet Union showed patients with chronic heart failure benefited greatly from taking Ginger. Japanese researchers have also found that fresh or powdered Ginger lowers blood pressure while stimulating the circulatory system.

Fresh Ginger juice has been shown to lower serum glucose levels in animals by assisting the body in assimilation and metabolism of sugar. Ginger also helps regulate blood sugar by increasing digestion and helping the body tap into its energy stores.

A key ingredient in a variety of European digestive aids, Ginger root contains the digestive enzyme zingibain. It also stimulates the production of saliva and tones the intestines. This is important for people with congestive heart failure as poor blood flow leads to sluggish digestion and gastrointestinal discomfort.

Part of the daily diet in hot, humid countries such as India, Ginger aids digestion and helps preserve food. In the West, Ginger is used to flavor a variety of foods ranging from Ginger Ale to Ginger Snaps.

A love of marmalade led Dr. Charles Dorso of Cornell University Medical College to discover that Ginger helps prevent the formation of clots in the bloodstream.

Dorso was using his own platelet blood cells as the "normal control" in an experiment when he noticed his blood wasn't coagulating as it normally did. Then he recalled the night before he had indulged to excess in a tasty marmalade called "Ginger and Grapefruit." Ginger makes up 15 percent of the ingredients in the jelly.

To test his theory, Dorso mixed a bit of powdered Ginger with samples of his colleagues' blood. The platelets refused to stick together even after he added large amounts of a substance that stimulates blood clotting. The Cornell researchers theorize that it is Gingerol in the Ginger that acts as a natural anti-coagulant or blood thinner.

Ginger can be combined with other heart herbs as a tonic, a stimulant and an efficient delivery herb. It can be eaten fresh or sipped as an infusion using one teaspoon of fresh root or 1½ teaspoons powdered root. Ginger can also be used in a compress with Cayenne to stimulate circulation in the veins.

Mowrey's circulation formula combines Ginger root with Cayenne, Kelp, Gentian root and Blue Vervain to supplement his cardiac tonic or blood pressure blends. He suggests 2-3 capsules per day. He also mixes Ginger with Cayenne, Siberian Ginseng, Gotu Kola, Kelp and Peppermint leaves to combat fatigue that plagues those with heart failure and build back strength and stamina.

Ginkgo (Latin name: *Ginkgo Biloba*)

Next to the Dinglin Temple near Shandong, China stands a

3,000-year-old specimen of this amazing tree whose leaves have provided relief for a myriad of ailments. A natural vasodilator, Ginkgo Biloba has been shown to be very effective in treating a variety of conditions that arise from diminished cardiac and cerebral circulation due to congestive heart failure.

By boosting cerebral circulation, Ginkgo Biloba helps relieve confusion and preserve memory while increasing overall alertness and the ability to concentrate. By stimulating peripheral circulation, the herb alleviates the CHF patient's hyper-sensitivity to the cold and eases cramping in the legs caused by insufficient blood supply to the muscles.

Unlike conventional vasodilator drugs, Ginkgo Biloba does not sacrifice cerebral circulation for peripheral blood flow. Ginkgo stimulates peripheral, cerebral and vascular blood flow; feeding the heart, muscles, organs, brain and central nervous system.

As a neurological tonic, Ginkgo stabilizes neural membranes, maintains proper electrolyte balance, normalizes neurological transmitter functions and removes metabolic toxins.

Ginkgo stimulates the production of neurotransmitters critical to the proper contraction of the heart and blood vessels throughout the body. It also reactivates beta receptors that dilate the peripheral blood vessels and open airways in the lungs.

In patients with high blood pressure, Ginkgo Biloba prevents breaches in the brain-blood barrier that would allow toxins to be passed from blood vessels to the brain cells. By safeguarding the brain-blood barrier, Ginkgo diminishes swelling due to cerebral edema (fluid retention) which may restore proper brain function in patients with severe CHF.

Extracts of Ginkgo Biloba leaf have been used in China for over 5,000 years to treat disorders of the lung and heart. Outside China, Ginkgo is contained in an Ayurvedic elixir called Soma and a concentrated extract called Tebonin used in Europe and Mexico for treatment of circulatory problems. Ginkgo Biloba has few side effects but it could take weeks or months before patients feel significant improvement.

Ginkgo Biloba leaf contains flavoglycosides, proanthro-cyanides bioflavonoids and a unique substance called ginkgolides which acts as an antioxidant and keeps platelets from sticking together to form blood clots that could lead to heart attack or stroke. Bioflavonoids, also considered antioxidants, strengthen the capillary walls and increase absorption of vitamin C.

Studies show ginkgolide B, a healing substance found only in Ginkgo Biloba, may prevent the body from rejecting transplanted organs. This is especially important for patients with end-stage CHF seeking a heart transplant.

While Ginkgo Biloba is not considered a hypotensive herb, it may help prevent high blood pressure. Ginkgo stimulates prostanoids in the body. Prostanoids dilate blood vessels, keeping blood pressure lower.

Extensive tests were performed on Ginkgo in Europe to determine potential side-effects before the herb was approved for consumption. In rare cases, people have developed nausea, headache or skin rash that appears to be an allergic reaction. However, Ginkgo is non-toxic even in high doses.

Extracted, concentrated Ginkgo Biloba containing 24 percent bioflavoniods, 24 percent flavoglycosides, 10 percent quercetin (a flavonoid), ginkgolides and bilobilides is the form most commonly used in studies showing the herb's effectiveness. The usual dosage in 40 clinical studies performed since 1975 was 120 milligrams of extract per day.

Ginkgo Biloba can be taken alone or with other herbs as a therapeutic tonic. The standard clinically recommended dosage is 40 milligrams of the dried herb taken 3 times daily, according to Hoffmann.

Hoffmann's cardiac tonic formula for CHF mixes 1 part Ginkgo Biloba with 3 parts Hawthorn, and 1 part each of Linden Blossom, Dandelion leaf, Motherwort and Cramp Bark.

Gotu Kola (Latin name: *Centella Asiatica*)

Considered a brain food, Gotu Kola also rejuvenates the heart and has been prescribed by herbalists as a treatment for congestive heart failure.

Gotu Kola contains medicinal properties that help lower blood pressure by dilating peripheral blood vessels, neutralize blood acids, act as a diuretic to rid the body of excess water and ease fatigue by stimulating blood flow. It purifies the blood while soothing the nerves.

Gotu Kola is high in heart-sustaining nutrients like magnesium, calcium and vitamin A (beta carotene). A neural and glandular tonic, Gotu Kola is not related to Kola Nut and does not contain caffeine.

Hailed as veritable Fountain of Youth, Gotu Kola is said to delay aging and cure senility. Its popularity spawned the Indian proverb "A leaf or two a day will keep old age away."

This creeping plant with the fan-shaped leaves has long been used in China and India to promote longevity, boost brain power, heal wounds and cure nervous disorders. Gotu Kola stimulates the transmission of nerve impulses, enhancing brain function through the central nervous system.

Gotu Kola is a safe herb and has no side effects even in high doses. A tea can be made using one ounce of herb per pint of water. Drink one half cup of tea three times a day. Taken as a powdered extract, the recommended dosage is 60-120 mgs. per day. The tincture dosage is 15-30 drops three times per day.

Author Daniel Mowrey made Gotu Kola a key ingredient in another tonic to treat CHF symptoms and causes such as cardiac insufficiency, high blood pressure and atherosclerosis.

Mowrey's circulatory blend mixes equal parts of Gotu Kola, Bilberry, Butcher's Broom and Ginger Root. He recommends taking 1-2 capsules a day for prevention, 2-4 capsules a day to treat acute conditions and 1-4 capsules per day for long-term treatment of chronic conditions.

Valerian (Latin name: *Valeriana Officinalis*)

The most cited sedative in herbal pharmacopoeia, Valerian is best know for its soothing effect on the nervous system. However, the aromatic herb also has a calming effect on the circulatory system as it slows the action of the heart while increasing the force of each beat, quiets heart palpitation and lowers high blood pressure.

With a smell like dirty sweat socks, the mild tasting herb may not be as appetizing as it is effective. Valerian is considered one of the most useful herbs for treating heart palpitations and arrhythmias that can be either the cause or the result of congestive heart failure.

By relaxing the tension created by the demands of modern life, Valerian also helps keep blood pressure low and contributes to the overall health of the heart and circulatory system. Experiments on animals have shown Valerian can prevent the onset of cardiac insufficiency – the beginnings of heart failure.

For those who already have CHF, Valerian also targets emotional and mental disturbances that come with such a chronic debilitating condition. It relieves tension, worry, nervousness, headache and irritability and relaxes cramping muscles. It grants a good night sleep to those who need it most without morning grogginess or fear of addiction.

Hundreds of experiments have been conducted on Valerian in Germany and Russia substantiating the herb's effectiveness in the treatment of circulatory, nervous and digestive system disorders as well as insomnia.

In one study, a group of men with high blood pressure drank a glass of water with Valerian extract. Physical examinations of the subjects revealed Valerian had a general tranquilizing effect. This was supported by Electroencephalogram (EEG) readings showing an elective neurotropic action in higher brain centers which indicates mild sedation. EEG tests record electrical activity in the brain.

Valmane, a German drug containing pure Valerian root, is commonly prescribed in Europe to treat hyperactivity, anxiety and insomnia. In Guatemala, Valerian is a key ingredient in a commonly used herbal blood pressure medication.

Even in high doses, Valerian and Valmane were shown to have no side effects or toxicity, unlike the drugs commonly prescribed to treat emotional disturbances, behavioral problems, psychosomatic illnesses and nervous disorders.

As a sedative, muscle relaxant and pain reliever, Valerian

allays minor aches and grants a deep natural sleep without lingering drowsiness. In fact, the herb improves coordination, increases concentration and boosts energy levels according to a series of studies on animals and humans.

It seems a paradox that Valerian can improve physical coordination and mental concentration while slowing overall motor activity. As an ideal tonic for the nervous system, Valerian merely soothes the erratic pitches of tension, allowing the system to function smoothly and more efficiently.

As a case in point, in a German experiment 120 children with behavioral disorders were given Valmane. Over a period of several weeks, the Valerian-based drug calmed hyperactivity and anxiety in over 75 percent of the children allowing them to concentrate on the task at hand.

Valerian does not interact with alcohol so there is no resulting depression or the dangerous synergism associated with tranquilizers such as Valium. Over time, taking synthetic sedatives like Valium can result in addiction and loss of locomotor coordination. Herbalists recommend using Valerian to safely ween patients off Valium.

While easing stress and assuring a good night's sleep, studies show Valerian also slows the heart rate while increasing the power of each beat, making the action of the heart more efficient and less strained. By quieting heart palpitations (arrhythmias) and lowering blood pressure, Valerian can help prevent CHF or at least slow its progress.

Besides the benefits Valerian brings to the circulatory and nervous systems, it also aids digestion. By stimulating the secretion of gastrointestinal juices, Valerian enhances the function of a sluggish digestive system.

Used as both a perfume and a condiment since the 11th century, Valerian is a rich source of calcium. It is also high in magnesium, chromium and iron.

Valerian root should not be boiled since it is the essential oils that contain most of the therapeutic properties of the herb. It can be taken as a tea, added to liquids as an extract or ingested in powered capsule form.

An infusion ensures none of the precious volatile oils are lost. Use 2 teaspoons of dried Valerian for each cup of hot water. To make a cold infusion, pour a glass of cold water over 2 teaspoons of root and let stand for 8-10 hours.

The tincture dosage is 1/2 to 2 teaspoons taken as

needed (up to 3 teaspoonfuls in a short period of time).
Caution should be observed when using Valerian extracts
and tinctures.

Although overdose is rare, using the concentrated forms
of the herb makes it possible to reach the high amounts necessary. Symptoms of overdose include headache, muscle
spasms, depression or anxiety. Cut back on the dosage and
symptoms will disappear completely.

Combining Valerian with Gentian and Peppermint is
said to boost its effectiveness as a cardiac tonic. Hawthorn
and Valerian are commonly paired to treat arrhythmia
although Dr. Christopher recommended an infusion of
Cayenne pepper and Valerian to treat palpitations. Mixing
Valerian with Hops and Passion Flower can dispose of even
the most stubborn insomnia.

Rosemary (Latin name: *Rosmarinus Officinalis*)

A mild circulatory stimulant, Rosemary calms
irritated nerves and soothes an upset stomach.
The leaf and twig of this aromatic herb also
encourage cell growth and repair.

Rosemary is high in minerals critical to
proper heart function including easily-assimil-
able calcium, magnesium, phosphorus, potassium and sodium. The herb helps the body
maintain the proper electrolyte balance needed for a strong, steady heart rhythm and a
healthy nervous system.

Used since ancient times to lower blood pressure, Rosemary also strengthens the capillaries,
boosting the overall health of the circulatory system.

German physicians prescribe Rosemary to
recover energy lost during long convalescence. A
tonic for both the circulatory and the nervous system, Rosemary is also employed to ease depression brought on by
debilitating illnesses like congestive heart failure.

Used in China as a headache cure, smooth muscle stimulant and stomach ache remedy, the oil contained in the herb
appears to have a calming effect on nerves and muscles.

A staple in herbal folklore and culinary history,
Rosemary is considered a very safe herb unless taken in

excess. It should be used as one part of a total therapy to prevent or treat congestive heart failure.

Rosemary can be taken alone up to three times a day in a tincture dosage of 1-2 milliliters or a cup of infusion (tea), according to herbalist and author David Hoffmann. However, it's best used in a cardiac tonic formula such as in Mowrey's mixture described previously.

Like Garlic, Onion, Cayenne and other culinary herbs, adding a pinch of Rosemary to the diet will do more than just spice up the meal.

Black Cohosh (Latin name: *Cimicifuga Racemosa*)

Black Cohosh was introduced to herbal medicine by the American Indians as Squaw Root – a reference to its use in the treatment of uterine problems.

While researching the root's effectiveness in regulating menstruation, relieving labor pain and promoting quick and uncomplicated delivery, scientists discovered the benefits of Black Cohosh for the circulatory and nervous systems.

Black Cohosh is a natural vasodilator and cardiac stimulant. It lowers blood pressure and reduces the heart rate while increasing the force of each beat. One experiment using Black Cohosh extract produced a significant drop in blood pressure which was attributed to active, water soluble resin in the herb.

According to studies in Europe, Black Cohosh works on the circulatory system through the central nervous system, relaxing smooth muscles and nerves. Studies show it decreases the vasomotor reflexes that close and open the carotid arteries. By slowing these reflexes of the central nervous system, the herb dilates the arteries and lowers blood pressure. It also dilates the peripheral blood vessels, equalizing circulation throughout the body.

One of the most common ingredients in herbal medicine, Black Cohosh also aids digestion and acts as a diuretic by stimulating the kidneys and liver. Aside from soothing cramps, Black Cohosh routes rheumatism pain and eases the discomfort of arthritis. As an expectorant Black Cohosh has been used to treat bronchitis and other chronic pulmonary ailments.

For heart palpitations or high blood pressure, Dr.

Christopher recommends taking one teaspoonful of Black Cohosh infusion every 30 minutes or three teaspoons every hour. Cut back on the dosage if you become nauseous as it may indicate overdose.

Black Cohosh can be added to other cardiac tonic mixtures or taken alone. Mowrey recommends a high blood pressure tonic consisting of equal parts of Black Cohosh, Garlic, Valerian, Cayenne and Kelp. To lower blood pressure and regulate cholesterol, he recommends 2-3 capsules 3-4 times per day. To prevent high blood pressure and supplement his cardiac tonic blend detailed earlier, he suggests 3-5 capsules per day.

The antispasmodic properties of Black Cohosh dissolve more completely in alcohol than in water. Those effects may be more powerful in a tincture than an infusion. Add 15-30 drops of tincture to one cup of water.

Prickly Ash (Latin name: *Zanthoxylum Americanum*)

As a cardiac stimulant, Prickly Ash is slower to take effect than Cayenne but its effects are more long-lasting. The bark or berries of the plant increase circulation and remove obstructions in the blood stream.

Prickly Ash stimulates the lymphatic system, digestive system and the mucous membranes as well as the circulatory system. It acts as a whole body tonic, warming the extremities, healing wounds, aiding digestion and purifying the blood. As a diuretic and cardiac stimulant, Prickly Ash has been used to treat edema that results from congestive heart failure.

Used to treat a wide range of ailments including rheumatism, cholera, gonorrhea, ulcers and liver ailments, Prickly Ash was included in the *U.S. Pharmacopoeia* for over 100 years.

With its wide-reaching benefits, Prickly Ash makes an effective delivery herb. As an ingredient in tonic formulas, it speeds the herbs where they need to go. It can be combined with other cardiac tonic ingredients in a capsule, tea or tincture.

If taken by itself, an infusion of Prickly Ash made from 1-2 teaspoons of dried bark or berries can be drunk three times a day. A strong decoction is made by boiling 1 ounce of bark in 3 pints of water until only one pint remains. The decoction should be taken in small, frequent doses totaling two cups a day.

Dr. Christopher suggests a blood purifier which can be made by combining 1/2 ounce of Prickly Ash bark, 1/2 ounce Guaiac resin, 1/2 ounce Buckbean herb and six fresh pods of Cayenne pepper. Simmer for 15 minutes in a tightly covered container and cool in the sealed pot to preserve essential oils. Drink one wine glass full three times a day.

Cramp Bark (Latin name: *Viburnum Opulus*)

As the name implies, Cramp Bark's main use is for menstrual cramps, but the herb works for spasms of any kind including heart palpitations. Known as Guelder Rose, Cramp Bark was used in England to treat palpitations, heart disease and rheumatism. Since it's mildly hypotensive, it can also help regulate blood pressure. High blood pressure and arrythmias are both causes and symptoms of congestive heart failure.

As an anti-spasmodic and nerve tonic, Cramp Bark has been used to treat muscle spasms from the uterus to the heart, soothe the nervous system, ease asthma attacks and prevent miscarriages.

Seldom taken alone, Cramp Bark is usually part of a blend, lending its antispasmodic properties to treatments for monthly pain and rheumatism or cardiac tonic blends such as Hoffmann's heart failure formula described previously (Hawthorn, Ginkgo, Linden Blossom, Dandelion leaf, Motherwort).

As a hypotensive herb, Cramp Bark can also be found in formulas to lower blood pressure. Hoffmann's hypertension tonic combines 1 part Cramp Bark with 2 parts Hawthorn, 1 part Linden Blossom, 1 part Yarrow and 1 part Valerian. It can be taken as an alcohol-based tincture (1 teaspoon three times a day) or as an infusion (2 teaspoons in a cup of boiling water three times a day).

A decoction of Cramp Bark alone can be made by boiling 2 teaspoons of bark in a pint of water. Take one teaspoon as needed.

Linden Blossom/Lime Flower
(Latin name: *Tilia Europea*)

The dried flowers of the Linden Blossom
are used to ease nervous tension and lower
blood pressure. The sweet-smelling herb
reduces the strain on the circulatory system
while ridding the body of excess water.

A favorite sedative in folk medicine since the Middle
Ages, it is said just the fragrance of Linden Blossom soothes
the soul, relieves worries and causes drowsiness.

As a cardiac tonic, Linden Blossom is thought to help
prevent atherosclerosis and high blood pressure from developing – two causes of congestive heart failure. It is also used
to treat elevated blood pressure caused by nervous tension.

While there is little scientific research available on the
effectiveness of Linden Blossom, it is listed in the *British
Herbal Pharmacopoeia* as a treatment for high arterial pressure and vascular headaches.

An infusion can made from one teaspoonful of dried
blossoms per cup of water. Drink one cupful, warm not hot,
before bedtime as a sedative and a cardiac tonic for edema
and high blood pressure.

Hoffmann considers Linden Blossom an essential ingredient in his cardiac tonic formula for CHF which mixes 1
part Linden Blossom with 3 parts Hawthorn and 1 part each
of Ginkgo, Dandelion leaf, Motherwort and Cramp Bark.

Herbalist Daniel Mowrey cautions that frequent, long-
term use of Linden Blossom tea (infusion) has been linked
to possible heart damage. However, smaller, therapeutic
doses in capsule form are nontoxic, he said. Mixed with
other herbs in a cardiac tonic formula, Linden Blossom is
both safe and effective.

STIMULATING, STRENGTHENING SEDATIVES

Hops (Latin name: *Humulus Lupulus*)

Hops stimulates circulation while relaxing the nervous system. The flowers or cones increase the heart's pumping
action and boost capillary circulation, reduce inflammation
of the liver, increase the flow of urine, purify the blood and

relax the central nervous system. These are all benefits of great use to CHF patients.

As a tonic, Hops eases heart palpitation, cleanses the blood and increases the flow of urine by toning the liver and gallbladder. A gentle diuretic with a spicy smell and bitter flavor, Hops also soothes the bladder.

Used primarily to treat nervous disorders, Hops is such an effective sedative, just laying your head on a pillow filled with Hops is said to end insomnia, dispell delirium, calm anxiety, relax tensions and ease earache.

King George III used a Hops pillow to cure his insomnia but it can also be taken internally with no side effects or lingering drowsiness. Studies show it takes only 20-40 minutes after drinking Hops tea for the patient to feel a calm come over them. Hops targets the kind of overwrought anxious sleeplessness CHF patients suffer.

In the U.S., Hops has been used primarily in the production of beer. However, it is also a common ingredient in herbal sleep aids. In Europe, Hops has been used successfully to treat a variety of sleep disorders.

High in B vitamins, Hops also improves appetite, soothes liver ailments and eases stomach distress. Its antispasmodic principles quell gastric distress and intestinal spasms while its sedative properties calm the nerves.

Recommended dosage is either half a cup of an infusion made from half an ounce of the dried flowers to one pint of hot water or 1-2 milliliters of Hops tincture three times a day.

A nighttime sleep tonic can by made by mixing equal parts of Hops, Passion Flower and Valerian. One teaspoon in a cup of hot water should be taken shortly before bedtime.

Passion Flower (Latin name: *Passiflora Incarnata*)

Popular in Europe as a sedative and cardiac tonic, Passion Flower induces sleep gently so patients awaken refreshed.

Besides easing the insomnia that plagues those who suffer from congestive heart failure, Passion Flower also has been used in Germany to treat cardiovascular neurosis and weak circulation. As a hypotensive, it lowers blood pressure and helps prevent tachycardia – rapid heart beat.

Experiments on animals show chemicals in Passion Flower dilate coronary arteries, which may account for its effectiveness in lowering blood pressure and boosting circulation.

In Germany, more than 50 preparations containing Passion Flower are available – some with Hawthorn and Valerian. Most are sedatives, but a portion are cardiac tonics. They are prescribed to treat such conditions as coronary artery disease, weak circulation, hyperactivity, asthma and cardiovascular neurosis.

Discovered in 1569 growing in the Peruvian mountains, the white flowers with purple-tinged petals were first used by the Indians to ease aches, relax muscle spasms and heal wounds.

Listed in the *U.S. Dispensary* for its ability to relieve insomnia and certain types of spasmodic disorders, Passion Flower grows wild in the Southern United States, producing edible fruit the size of a chicken egg.

Numerous studies have shown Passion Flower is not addictive and has no lingering effects – unlike narcotic sedatives. It induces a natural sleep with easy breathing and no mental depression or confusion. Herbalists recommend it for helping wean patients off prescription tranquilizers.

One cupful of an infusion made from 1/2 to 1 teaspoonful of the dried herb can be drunk at bedtime to avoid sleeplessness. Tincture dosage is 15-60 drops or 1/4 to 1 teaspoon in water up to 3 times a day. Start with the lower dosage and increase as needed. Hoffmann suggests mixing Valerian, Passion Flower and Hops to ease nervous tension and quell insomnia.

It should be noted that Passion Flower (Passiflora Incarnata) is nontoxic and does not contain cyanide as once thought. A different ornamental species, Passiflora Caerulea, contains the poison. Check labels to be sure you're getting Passiflora Incarnata. Despite its reputation as an antispasmodic herb, Passion Flower is not recommended for use by pregnant women as it has been known to cause uterine contractions.

Peppermint (Latin name: *Mentha Piperita*)

Flavorful, aromatic and versatile, this popular herb relieves insomnia, strengthens heart muscles, quiets palpitations, aids digestion, quells nausea and dispels diarrhea.

A mild vasodilator, Peppermint clears circulatory congestion by stimulating blood flow. It helps assure a proper blood supply to the brain and clears congestion throughout the entire circulatory system. The fragrant leaf is high in vitamins and minerals essential for heart health including magnesium, calcium, potassium and vitamin A.

Peppermint is one of the best herbs for soothing ailments of the stomach and digestive system. Its volatile oils act as a mild anesthetic, numbing the stomach walls and easing nausea and intestinal pain. It relaxes smooth muscle spasms, stimulates the flow of digestive juices and the secretion of bile, tones the gastrointestinal system, dispels gas and stops diarrhea.

As an antibacterial herb, Peppermint kills more than 30 types of micro-organisms that can cause digestive and other problems. Studies have shown the herb rids the body of such "bugs" as scarlet fever, the Asian flu, Herpes Simplex, the mumps, rheumatic fever, pneumonia (Staphlococcus aureus), sinusitis and cystitis. It has also proven effective in the treatment of colds and flu.

As a nerve tonic, Peppermint strengthens and calms the nervous system, easing tension, relieving headache and boosting the ability to concentrate. As an added bonus, the volatile oils appear to stimulate the entire body. Used to treat fatigue, Peppermint imparts a feeling of renewed energy and vitality scientists have not yet been able to explain.

Used to flavor a variety of products ranging from toothpaste to candy canes, cough syrup to liquor, Peppermint is consumed around the world. Over a million cups of peppermint tea are drunk daily.

Cultivated in Europe since the 1700s, fields of the herb are now tended from the United States to Japan. Native to England, Peppermint can be found growing wild in the U.S., particularly near garbage dumps. Of the two varieties, White Peppermint is said to contain a higher concentration of the medicinal menthol oil than Black Peppermint.

The green leafy herb can be taken as a tea, infusion or extract but it should never be boiled as the healing power is contained in its delicate volatile oils. To make an infusion, pour a cup of boiling water over 1 teaspoonful of

Peppermint leaves, cover and steep for 10 minutes. Strain, sweeten and drink hot.

Since Peppermint tea is high in astringent tannic acids, it is advisable to add a little milk or cream to the tea to neutralize the tannins. Long-term, frequent ingestion of tea high in tannic acids has been linked to ailments such as cancer of the esophagus and liver damage. However, adding milk or cream was found to render tannic acids harmless.

Peppermint makes a good ingredient in a circulatory tonic and can be also added to other herbal mixtures to enhance their flavor while aiding digestion and assimilation.

Mowrey's anti-fatigue formula mixes Peppermint with Ginseng, Ginger, Gotu Kola, Kelp and Cayenne. He recommends a maintenance dose of 1-2 capsules per day and up to 6 capsules a day for acute conditions.

NOURISHING NORMALIZING HERBS

Kelp (Latin name: *Laminaria*)

Kelp nourishes the circulatory system, lowers blood pressure, invigorates a sluggish heartbeat and regulates the function of the thyroid gland. Proper functioning of the thyroid gland helps prevent atherosclerosis and congestive heart failure.

Located in the neck, the thyroid gland secretes hormones that control growth, trigger the onset of puberty, regulate metabolism, stimulate cellular activity and adjust the function of internal organs and tissues.

Thyroxine, the primary hormone secreted by the thyroid, is critical for the proper assimilation of vitamins, minerals and other nutrients. Thyroxine converts beta carotene to vitamin A, aids in absorption of carbohydrates and proper protein synthesis.

An overactive or hyperthyroid gland can lead to a condition called thyrotoxicosis. Characterized by rapid heart beat, enlarged glands, tremors and loss of weight, untreated thyrotoxicosis can lead to congestive heart failure and death.

Thyroid disease is virtually unknown in Japan where up to 25 percent of the diet is made up of Kelp. The large, flat-leaf frond aquatic plant grows in the Pacific Ocean at depths of 10-150 feet.

Kelp supplies the thyroid with iodine and other nutrients it needs to function properly. The thyroid needs a steady supply of iodine to regulate the body's metabolic rate. From the seawater in which it thrives, Kelp also pulls proteins, essential fatty acids, carbohydrates, potassium and heart-healthy trace minerals like magnesium.

Since a healthy thyroid helps the body burn fats that might otherwise collect in the arteries, Kelp can also play a part in preventing atherosclerosis – another cause of congestive heart failure. Kelp also contains Algin, a natural fiber which has proven cholesterol-lowering properties to keep the arteries clear.

A 1986 study showed that powdered Kelp fiber may prevent strokes. Scientists were feeding rats with high blood pressure excessive amounts of salt. The group of rats that also ate the powdered brown seaweed suffered no strokes while their fellow salt-eating vermin all had strokes. Powdered Kelp seemed to neutralize the excess sodium in the rats' diet, scientists reported.

While Kelp targets the thyroid, it also nourishes the heart and nervous system. A cardiac tonic high in essential nutrients for proper heart function, Kelp reduces stress on the heart by increasing its efficiency. It stimulates the heart gently and lowers blood pressure.

Experiments performed on frogs' hearts show Kelp increases contractile power in the atria. Kelp was found to contain fatty acids that stimulate the heart muscle and a histamine substance that speeds up atrial contractions in a sluggish heart.

High in oxygen, Kelp feeds tissues, organs and muscles deprived of oxygen by a malfunctioning heart.

In Japan, a healthy dose of the brown seaweed is served up in soup, salad, sauces and sushi. Kelp flavors jams and jellies. The sea-spawned flour is used to make noodles – one of the nation's favorite fast foods. Researchers theorize that Kelp consumption may account for the fact that the Land of the Rising Sun has few cases of heart disease, obesity, high blood pressure and thyroid dysfunction compared to Western nations.

Aside from their nourishing diet, the Japanese have a formula called Kombu made from Kelp that has been used for many years to treat high blood pressure. The results of recent studies support the tonic's effectiveness.

Kelp has no known toxicity or side-effects. Studies have shown the arsenic contained in the brown seaweed is completely indigestible and is harmlessly excreted. It should be noted, Kelp is a general term for brown seaweed – particularly the Laminaria species. Ascophyllum and Macrocystis species have also been used.

Kelp can be added to the diet or taken in capsules alone or in a variety of formulas. Mowrey's cardiac tonic formula mixes Kelp with Hawthorn, Cayenne, Motherwort and Rosemary. His high blood pressure blend combines Kelp with Garlic, Valerian, Black Cohosh and Cayenne. (See Garlic.) He also adds Kelp to his diuretic, detoxification and anti-fatigue formulas. (See Ginger.)

Gentian Root (Latin name: *Gentiana Lutea*)

Gentian Root makes a bitter tonic known to normalize the function of the thyroid gland, stimulate circulation and aid the digestion and assimilation of nutrients.

Considered one of the best strengthening herbs, the root of this yellow-flowered plant is high in heart nourishing minerals like magnesium. The roots also store a large supply of revitalizing oxygen.

Famed herbalist Nicholas Culpepper said of bitter European Gentian Root, "It comforts the heart and protects it against faintings and swoonings."

Recommended for exhausted travelers and bedridden convalescents, Gentian Root restores energy and rebuilds an ailing constitution. Gentian Root stimulates the sluggish circulation of the CHF sufferer. By assuring the digestive organs receive a sufficient amount of blood, Gentian enables the body to assimilate more nutrients to feed all the organs.

Gentian promotes the production of bile, saliva and gastric juices; emptying the stomach more rapidly and replenishing nutrients more reliably in patients with sluggish circulation.

Named after King Gentius, ancient ruler of Illyria, Gentian Root grows in the mountainous areas of Europe from the Black Forest to the Pyrenees. Used in Germany and Switzerland in an alcoholic drink, Gentian Root also can be taken as a tea, a tincture, an infusion or a powder.

Chewing the root kills smokers' craving for cigarettes, according to herbal lore.

A decoction made from 1/2 teaspoon of peeled root can be sipped warm shortly before meals. An infusion can be made from 1 teaspoon of powered herb per cup of hot water. Tincture dosage is 1-2 milliliters three times a day. Extremely high doses can cause gastrointestinal distress.

As a bitter tonic for the circulatory system, Hoffmann suggests combining Gentian root with Valerian and Hops. Christopher recommends a revitalizing tonic made by steeping 1 ounce of Gentian Root, 1 ounce of Peruvian Bark, 1 ounce of Dandelion Root and 1 ounce of Bitter Orange peel for half an hour in 1½ pints of water. Strain and add three ounces of brandy. He recommends a maintenance dose of one teaspoonful taken with meals.

Sarsaparilla (Latin name: *Similax Officinalis*)

A blood-purifier, Sarsaparilla contains traces of magnesium sulfate which acts as a gentle laxative; sulfur which keeps food from putrefying in the intestines; iron to help oxygenate the blood; calcium oxalate which boosts the oxygen level while absorbing carbon dioxide; potassium chloride which rids the body of clot-causing fibrin; and magnesium which tones the heart muscle, improves contraction and protects against heart disease, congestive heart failure and other ailments.

The red root is also said to contain testosterone, progesterone and cortin. Studies show Sarsaparilla boosts testosterone activity and aids the functioning of the body as a whole. The hormone testosterone is said to be the natural steroid of body builders – necessary for toning, strengthening and developing muscle tissue.

Besides balancing hormone levels, Sarsaparilla purifies the blood, cleanses the system of infections and helps cure skin problems such as eczema and psoriasis. Antibiotic principles contained in the root neutralize microbial substances in the blood stream, protecting the body from infection.

As a cardiac tonic, the root boosts circulation and removes obstructions from the bloodstream. It also acts as a diuretic, stimulating the flow of urine and easing edema. It heals liver inflammations and eases the pain of chronic rheumatism.

The benefits of Sarsaparilla as a total body tonic may be due to its ability to remove toxins from the cells, blood stream and glands. Accumulation of wastes interferes with the delivery of nutrients, weakening the body. By cleansing the entire body of wastes, Sarsaparilla refreshes and revitalizes the system. This is particularly important for convalescents and people suffering from chronic illnesses such as congestive heart failure.

Sarsaparilla's ability to cure a variety of ailments and invigorate the entire body was no surprise to the Amazon Indians. Swedish anthropologist Alfred Metraus found the Indians using Sarsaparilla long before their Northern counterparts. Hunting parties would go for long periods of time eating only Sarsaparilla root. The leaves and berries were used as an antidote for poison.

In the 1800s, Sarsaparilla root came into vogue in the United States as a spring tonic taken to eliminate toxins accumulated over the long winter. The root later reached greater heights of popularity as a flavoring for cookies, candy and beverages such as root beer.

In the War of 1812, Sarsaparilla was used to treat syphilis among the soldiers, proving to be more effective than mercury-based medicines without the chemical's harsh side effects. A Chinese study reported success rates of 90 percent in treating the venereal disease.

Sarsaparilla is usually mixed with other herbs to enhance their effectiveness and boost the overall health of the body. As a tonic for the nerves, blood and glands, Sarsaparilla can be added to previous cardiac tonic formulas to detoxify the body and support the other herbs in strengthening a weakened heart.

Dr. Christopher recommends a blood purifier made from an ounce each of Sarsaparilla root, Burdock, Guaiac chips, Cleavers, Fumitory and Licorice Root simmered in $3\frac{1}{2}$ quarts boiling water until one quart of liquid has been steamed away. Dosage is 1/2 cup three to four times a day.

Dosage of solely Sarsarparilla root is 1-2 milliliters of tincture or a cup of decoction made with 1-2 teaspoons of root three times a day.

Alfalfa (Latin name: *Medicago Sativa*)

A member of the legume family, Alfalfa is a diuretic known for its ability to lower cholesterol while boosting overall health. One of the most nutritious herbs, Alfalfa is high in vitamins A (beta carotene), D, E, B_1, B_{12}, B-6, and K.

A good source of protein and fiber, Alfalfa contains minerals essential to heart health including calcium, magnesium, iron, potassium, phosphorous, chlorophyll, niacin, zinc, biotin, folic acid, pantothenic acid, saponins and a host of digestive enzymes to assist in system delivery.

With all its nutrients balanced for complete absorption, Alfalfa helps to maintain or regain health. It nourishes the circulatory, glandular and nervous systems. It also stimulates the growth of connective tissue cells.

A diuretic and digestive aid, Alfalfa has been used to relieve edema. Its high fiber content aids digestion and removes toxins. The digestive enzymes contained in the plant help the body assimilate essential nutrients and sugars, and oxygenate the blood.

Hailed by Ancient Arabs as the "Father of All Foods," Alfalfa leaves are eaten as a vegetable in Russia while in the U.S., Alfalfa sprouts are more commonly consumed.

Studied for years, due in part to its importance to the livestock industry, Alfalfa's use by humans has primarily been to enhance other herbal formulas. Formulas commonly contain about 10 percent Alfalfa to boost nutrition and assist in delivery of the other herbs to the targeted areas of the body.

On its own, Alfalfa has been shown to be a primary ingredient for lowering cholesterol levels. One study showed Alfalfa saponins inhibited the normal rise in blood cholesterol levels as much as 25 percent in a test group of monkeys, rats and rabbits that was being fed a high cholesterol diet.

Alfalfa saponins are thought to lower cholesterol through the production of bile acids. Bile acids are needed to absorb cholesterol so it passes harmlessly out of the body.

Other studies have shown that besides lowering cholesterol and boosting nutrition, Alfalfa is also antibacterial and can rid the digestive system of carcinogenic chemicals. The herb initiates a complex cellular activity that neutralizes dietary carcinogens that build up in the small intestine and liver.

Like Sarsaparilla, Alfalfa is a whole body tonic that works best as a nutritious addition to herbal combinations. Mowrey suggests a whole body tonic consisting of equal parts of Sarsaparilla root, Alfalfa, Siberian Ginseng, Fo-ti, Saw Palmetto berries, Licorice Root, Kelp and Cayenne.

This mixture, according to Mowrey, will boost vitality, increase resistance to disease and support recovery from debilitating illnesses like congestive heart failure. The "ultimate tonic," this recipe touches every part of the body – veins, nerves, muscles, glands, arteries, organs, bones and of course, the heart. He recommends 2-12 capsules per day, taken as needed. Convalescents should take the maximum dosage.

Fo-ti (Latin name: *Polygonum Multiflorum, Ho-shou-wu*)

In China, Fo-ti is one of the most popular anti-aging herbs. A rejuvenating whole body tonic, Fo-ti has been used for hundreds of years to treat coronary artery disease, insomnia, cancer, fatigue, liver ailments and constipation.

As a cardiac tonic, Fo-ti lowers harmful cholesterol levels, regulates blood pressure and helps prevent atherosclerosis. Although little research has been done on Fo-ti in the West, scientists theorize that its benefits are derived from a substance called leucoanthrocyanidins (LAC).

Plants of a similar species containing LAC have been shown to act as vasodilators, opening up peripheral blood vessels; anti-coagulants, keeping clots from forming in the bloodstream; and hypotensives, regulating blood pressure. These are the same medicinal actions for which Fo-ti is renowned. Although LAC has not yet been isolated in Fo-ti, this would explain why the root works the way it does.

Fo-ti helps the body retain its youth by strengthening the heart and protecting the circulatory system from the ravages of age. For this reason, Fo-ti has been included in this collection of herbs to help prevent congestive heart failure.

For those with heart failure, Fo-Ti's effectiveness as a

vasodilator can take some of the strain off the weakened heart. Lowering high blood pressure may also keep the condition from progressing. As a vitality tonic, Fo-Ti may help restore some of the energy depleted by fighting chronic heart failure.

Fo-ti is said to be the herbal secret of longevity. Legend has it that Chinese herbalist Li Chung Yun lived to the ripe old age of 256 by daily ingestion of a formula containing Fo-ti and Ginseng.

Intrigued by the tale, Professor Menier of Paris experimented with the herb and isolated a substance he called Vitamin X. Vitamin X, according to Menier, rejuvenates brain cells, nerves and the endocrine glands. His results were verified by French biochemist Jules Lepine. Fo-ti also aids digestion and boosts metabolism of vitamins, minerals and nutrients.

Fo-Ti can be combined with other herbs to help resist disease or restore health such as Mowrey's Whole Body Tonic described in the section on Alfalfa.

An effective alcohol-based preparation which blends Fo-Ti and other oriental herbs is available in Chinese herb stores under the name "shou wu chih," according to herbalist Michael Tierra, author of *The Way of Herbs*.

Ginseng (Latin name: *Panax Ginseng, Eleutherococcus Senticosus, Panax Quinquefolius*)

The most commonly prescribed herb for fatigue in the Far East, Ginseng can help the body shrug off stress and increase the stamina of a failing heart so that it can withstand the extra workload.

The Chinese have been using Korean Ginseng (Panax Ginseng) for over 3,000 years to stimulate the circulatory and nervous systems, boost metabolism and regulate blood pressure and blood sugar.

Coming from the same botanical family, the three most common Ginsengs: Korean (Panax Ginseng), Siberian (Eleutherococcus Senticosus) and American (Panax Quinquefolius); all share medicinal similarities.

First mentioned in the *Shennong Herbal*, written before

the second century B.C., modern studies found that Ginseng works by helping the body "adapt" to the effects of stress.

The term "adaptogen" was coined for Ginseng by Russian scientist I.I. Brekhman, Ph.D. An adaptogen, according to Brekhman, helps the body cope with emotional and physical stress by normalizing body functions.

In his 1969 study, Brekhman found that Soviet soldiers were able to run faster with less strain if they took Ginseng. The Ginseng regulated high blood pressure and normalized low blood sugar during intense physical activity.

Japanese studies in the 1970s showed Ginseng increased mental acuity. Rats fed Ginseng were able to perform their tasks more accurately and efficiently than their counterparts. Another Japanese study showed Ginseng helps the body metabolize cholesterol quickly, preventing LDL cholesterol from building up in the blood stream.

All three Ginsengs share these adaptogen qualities in different degrees. American Ginseng is the mildest. Korean Ginseng is the most stimulating. Siberian Ginseng is not a true Ginseng but its actions are so similar that it's classified as one. Eleutherosides, the active chemical in Siberian Ginseng, performs very much like the ginsenosides in American and Korean Ginseng.

Korean (Panax) Ginseng has been used in China for over 3,000 years to regulate blood pressure, stimulate circulation, prevent heart disease and treat congestive heart failure.

Korean Ginseng strengthens the heart muscle, suppresses arrhythmias, tones the entire circulatory system and boosts the synthesis of cholesterol, lowering the level in the blood stream to help prevent atherosclerosis. Modern Chinese doctors still prescribe Ginseng to treat patients in the early stages of congestive heart failure.

As a whole body tonic, Korean Ginseng restores normal function of various systems in the body. It regulates blood pressure, blood sugar levels, blood clotting agents and balances red and white blood cell count. It neutralizes disease-causing free radicals and helps the body recover from stress, surgery or the effects of debilitating illness.

Perhaps because it's the strongest of the three, Korean Ginseng carries extra precautions for side effects American and Siberian Ginseng do not share. Excessive doses of Korean Ginseng have been known to cause high blood pressure, headaches, nervousness, insomnia and diarrhea.

However, it is important to note, Korean Ginseng's link to high blood pressure is controversial. Author and herbalist Earl Mindell contends that the study published in the *Journal of the American Medical Association* which revealed these negative side-effects was flawed. In his book *Earl Mindell's Herb Bible*, Mindell points out that the subjects of the so-called "Ginseng Abuse Syndrome" study used caffeine and took all forms of Ginseng – and even injected it.

Meanwhile, a 1992 study performed at the University of Saarland in Homburg-Saar, Germany showed that high doses of a combination of Ginseng and Ginkgo Biloba lowered blood pressure.

The researchers used Gincosan, a European product containing 60 mg. Ginkgo Biloba and 100 mg. Ginseng on a group of 10 volunteers. The group taking the highest doses of Gincosan (120 mg. Ginkgo and 200 mg. Ginseng) experienced a decrease in both systolic and diastolic blood pressure and heart rate. The low dose group taking half the higher dosage experienced a drop in systolic blood pressure only.

Ginseng has long been considered a male tonic. In women, it can cause irregular menstruation and the growth of facial hair. It is not recommended for use by pregnant women. However, Ginseng is often recommended to treat menopausal symptoms since it is believed to increase estrogen levels. Milder Siberian and American Ginseng appear to have less side effects in women but are only recommended for short-term use (no more than 3 months).

Siberian Ginseng (Eleutherococcus Senticosus) is often prescribed to fight fatigue and the effects of nervous tension. Siberian Ginseng works through the glands and the nervous system to help the body "adapt" to stressful conditions. By stimulating and nourishing the adrenal glands, it influences the cardiovascular, nervous, immune, digestive and reproductive systems. It has been shown to increase the stamina of a weakened heart and relieve edema.

As an "adaptogen," Siberian Ginseng has been used to treat stress-related cardiovascular disease. Like Korean Ginseng, Siberian Ginseng regulates blood sugar, increases cerebral circulation, adds stamina, boosts the body's resistance to disease by strengthening the immune system and helps ease the effects of stress.

Grown primarily in Wisconsin, American Ginseng is the mildest of Ginseng. It was used by the American Indians to treat nausea but is now employed around the world as an adaptogen and a whole body tonic.

Like Korean Ginseng, the American variety also contains ginsenosides. It also increases stamina, reduces blood cholesterol, regulates blood sugar, enhances the immune system and helps the body cope with the effects of stress. Side effects to the milder stimulant are rare but insomnia and allergic reactions have been reported.

Ginseng can be taken alone or in a tonic with other cardiac herbs such as Hawthorn, Cayenne, Motherwort and Rosemary. Since the quality of Ginseng, particularly Korean, is often adulterated, care must be taken to get the purest kind available. Read the label carefully and look for reputable supplement companies.

Mowrey's Fatigue formula combines Siberian Ginseng with Cayenne, Gotu Kola, Peppermint leaves and Ginger root.

To build back physical strength and stamina stolen by debilitating illness such as congestive heart failure, he recommends 4-6 capsules per day. For therapeutic maintenance, he suggests 2-4 capsules per day.

Siberian Ginseng is also part of Mowrey's Whole Body Tonic discussed under Alfalfa. The blend mixes Siberian Ginseng with Sarsaparilla root, Alfalfa, Fo-ti, Saw Palmetto berries, Licorice Root, Kelp and Cayenne.

For stress-related high blood pressure, Hoffmann suggests a formula that combines 1 part each of Siberian Ginseng, Linden Blossom, Yarrow, Cramp Bark, Valerian and Scullcap with 2 parts Hawthorn. Taken as a tincture, the dosage is 1 teaspoon 3 times a day. To make an infusion, use 2 teaspoons to a cup and drink 3 times a day.

To help recover from a heart attack and prevent another, Hoffmann suggests a tonic comprised of 1 part Siberian Ginseng, 3 parts Hawthorn, 2 parts Ginkgo and 1 part Linden Blossom. The preparation and dosage are the same as his high blood pressure formula described above. As an adaptogen, Siberian Ginseng will help the survivor cope with stress that could either be the cause or the result of a heart attack.

If taken alone, the recommended dosage is one capsule

up to three times a day or 1-2 cups of infusion (tea) per day. Heart failure patients with high blood pressure may wish to consult a medical practioner before taking Korean Ginseng.

CARDIAC CRISIS HERBS

Foxglove (Latin name: *Digitalis Purpurea*)

Irish legend holds that the bright crimson spots on the bell-shaped Foxglove flower are a warning of the poison contained within. Given the Latin name of Digitalis in 1542 by famed German herbalist Leonhard Fuchs, Foxglove was only used externally to heal sores. Now, a drug made from the leaves is one of the most frequently prescribed oral medications for the treatment of congestive heart failure.

Foxglove (Digitalis) regulates pulse, strengthens the heartbeat and enhances each contraction. It eases the stress of an enlarged heart and increases the amount of blood that feeds the organ itself, building stamina through nourishment. In addition, it's a powerful diuretic targeting water retention resulting from a failing heart and compensating kidneys.

Foxglove leaves contain four important chemicals, three are cardiac stimulants and one is a cardiac depressant. The most powerful of the stimulants is digitoxin which is highly toxic, not water soluble and cumulative. Digitalin also is not water soluble, but it's less poisonous. The third cardiac stimulant, Digitalein, dissolves readily in water. Digitonin, the cardiac depressant, appears to exert little influence over the effects of Digitalis.

Although Digitalis is toxic, it's safer to use the pill form than the natural Foxglove leaf because the dosage is uniform and easier to control. It's harder to standardize the dosage of the natural plant because of variations in leaf size, shape and thickness. Consequently, the herb itself has fallen out of use.

Foxglove or Digitalis has the power to save or destroy. The level of the drug must be monitored constantly as it can accumulate and poison the system. Symptoms of a Digitalis overdose include heart arrhythmia and low blood pressure. Over time, Digitalis can cause the heart muscle to degenerate due to constant stimulation.

Taking the herb Hawthorn with the drug Digitalis will

complement the effects of the potent cardiac stimulant so that less of the toxic drug will be necessary to do the same job as before. Needing less Digitalis gives the patient more time before the drug can build to a toxic level in the body. Hawthorn also supports the work of Digitalis by providing more nourishment and oxygen to the stimulated muscle.

While Hawthorn can enhance and support the work of Digitalis, herbalists agree it cannot replace the drug in cases of severe congestive heart failure. Due to the poisonous nature of Foxglove (Digitalis) and the seriousness of congestive heart failure, extreme caution must be taken before altering the prescribed dosage in any way. Any changes should be made under the supervision of a medical professional.

Lily of the Valley (Latin name: *Convallaria Majalis*)

Listed in the Merck Index as a cardiotonic plant, Lily of the Valley is one of the few herbal alternatives to the drug Digitalis. As a cardiac tonic and diuretic, Lily of the Valley has long been a valued treatment for congestive heart failure.

Called "Ladder-to-Heaven" the medicinal properties of the broad-leafed green plant with nodding white bell-like flowers were first publicized by Fourth Century herbalist Apuleius in his book *Herbal*.

Considered less powerful than Foxglove (Digitalis), Lily of the Valley slows the erratic beat of the laboring heart while increasing the strength of each contraction.

Unlike Digitalis, Lily of the Valley is water soluble so it doesn't accumulate in the body. However, some studies have shown Lily of the Valley can be toxic in high doses and, as other medicinal herbs, it must be used with caution and the recommended dosage should be respected.

Herbalist Roy Upton characterized the Lily of the Valley toxicity studies as a misuse of the scientific method.

"Most of the concerns were raised by reductionist scientists who only look at the cardioactive constituents," Upton said. "They take out the cardiac glycosides, feed half a ton to a rat until it dies and say there's an overdose danger."

Although Lily of the Valley has since been re-approved for use and took its place again among the other herbs listed in the Merck Index, it had already fallen out of favor with herbalists in the United States. Most, Upton said, have forgotten how to use the powerful cardiac stimulant. In Europe, particularly England, Lily of the Valley has enjoyed a long, unbroken history of use.

In England, practitioners of herbal medicine used Lily of the Valley freely to treat a variety of ailments ranging from fever to ulcers. In World War I, it was used by British soldiers at the front to fight the effects of poisonous gas. In Germany, a popular wine was made by mixing the flowers with raisins.

Lily of the Valley is the key ingredient in author Dick Quinn's heart formula for congestive heart failure. The self-taught herbalist blends 60 percent Lily of the Valley with 30 percent Hawthorn, 15 percent Rosemary and 5 percent Cayenne.

Mrs. Maude Grieve, author of *A Modern Herbal*, recommends an infusion of 1/2 ounce Lily of the Valley steeped in 1 pint of boiling water taken by the tablespoon.

Cactus Flower or Night Blooming Cereus
(Latin name: *Cactus or Selenicereus Grandiflorus*)

Similar in action but stronger than Hawthorn, the stem and root of Cactus Grandiflorus are used as a cardiac stimulant. Weaker than Lily of the Valley, Cactus Grandiflorus mirrors the effects of Digitalis but is not a cumulative toxin. As a safer alternative, Cactus Grandiflorus has been used as a substitute for Digitalis.

To relieve cardiac conditions like congestive heart failure, kidney and bladder ailments and prostate problems, the American Indians drank a tea made from fresh Cactus Grandiflorus roots and stems. A decoction of the plant has been used as both a cardiac tonic and a diuretic.

Also called Sweet-Scented Cactus and Night Booming Cereus, Cactus Grandiflorus first garnered attention when homeopathic doctor R. Rubinin started using it to treat heart disease in Naples, Italy.

Native to the Southern United States, Mexico, the West Indies and Naples, Cactus Grandiflorus stimulates the action of the heart and helps relieve edema caused by congestive heart failure.

In Europe, herbalists use Cactus Grandiflorus or Night

Blooming Cereus to wean patients off Digitalis, according to herbalist Roy Upton, president of the American Herbalists Guild. However, as Upton advised, precautions must be taken when considering substituting Lily of the Valley or Night Blooming Cereus for Digitalis.

Any change in medication should be done under the careful supervision of a medical practitioner. The body learns to rely on powerful cardiac stimulants like Digitalis, Lily of the Valley and Cactus Grandiflorus – especially under crisis conditions like severe congestive heart failure. Even change for the better can be a shock to the system if not managed properly and could cause a serious setback.

Although it is not a cumulative toxin like Digitalis, Cactus Grandiflorus is a strong medicinal herb and must be used with caution. Overdose can have serious side effects including hallucinations, mental confusion and gastric distress.

Upton's cardic tonic mixture blends 2-3 parts Cactus Grandiflorus or Night Blooming Cereus with 4 parts Hawthorn, 1 part Motherwort and 2-3 parts specific cardiac tonic herbs determined by the severity of the condition and its symptoms. It can be taken as a tincture for severe CHF or as a syrup in less acute cases.

To make a Cactus Grandiflorus tincture or extract, herbalist Maude Grieve recommends using fresh plants full of acrid milky juice. As a dosage, she suggests 1/2 to 1 millileters of tincture or up to 1/2 millileter of extract. In addition to homemade concoctions, a couple of commercial blends containing Cactus Grandiflorus are available in health stores.

Strophanthus (Latin name: *Strophanus Hispidus*)

Discovered in the woodlands of East Africa by European explorers before the turn of the century, Strophanthus was transformed from an arrow poison to a highly effective heart medication.

Arrows tipped with the pulp of crushed Strophanthus seeds paralyzed the hunter's prey without poisoning the meat. Strophanthin, the active medicinal ingredient in Strophanthus seeds, is now used in Germany to treat congestive heart failure under the name G-Strophanthin or Strodival.

Listed in herbal source books an adjunct to Digitalis, Strophanthin increases circulation and also acts as a diuretic, reducing edema. Hawthorn will also enhance the effects of Strodival by nourishing the heart and feeding oxygen to the weakened heart muscle.

German practitioners have found Strophanthin reduces acid that builds up in the left ventricle as a result of heart failure. Strophanthin is one of the primary treatments for acidosis which, according to European theory, is the real cause of heart attack and coronary artery disease.

Like Digitalis, Strophanthin can be toxic and should be used under the supervision of a medical practioner. Unlike Digitalis, Strophanthin is not cumulative and is proven safe as long as the dosage is not exceeded.

Symptoms of overdose may include gastric distress and anxiety. The German product Strodival MR, a different formulation of G-Strophanthin, has shown to be easier to tolerate for patients prone to digestive disturbances.

At this writing, Strodival (G-Strophanthin) is not available in the U.S. However, it can be imported directly from the German manufacture with the prescription of a U.S. doctor. See "Medical Approaches to Heart Failure" for more information on the drug Strodival and how to procure it.

For the whole herb Strophanthus, Maude Grieve recommends a maximum dosage of 1/2 grain (.03 grams) per day. As a tincture, Grieve suggests 5 to 15 drops per day

HERBS FOR ANEURYSM

Bilberry (Latin name: *Vaccinium Myrtillus*)

Bilberry's ability to repair and restore leaky blood vessels and forestall atherosclerosis makes it a beneficial addition to the prevention and treatment of both congestive heart failure and aneurysm.

An aneurysm is formed when hard deposits of plaque (atherosclerosis) weaken the artery wall which is then pushed out by the pressure of blood flow. Bilberry restores elasticity to leaky, stiff, fragile capillaries that tend to break or distend. These leaky blood vessels lose essential fluids and nutrients before they get to the organs and tissues they are intended to feed.

By healing the blood vessels, Bilberry may be able to head off a variety of vascular disorders that can trigger congestive heart failure such as high blood pressure and atherosclerosis.

Recent studies show that not only does Bilberry restore a supple strength to the blood vessels, it also helps prevent hardening of the arteries by inhibiting the deposit of calcium plaque on the inside of the arteries.

A tonic for the entire circulatory system, Bilberry works by stimulating peripheral circulation and strengthening the capillaries. It also acts as a blood thinner and has been used to prevent strokes.

Most commonly used to treat vision problems, Bilberry improves blood supply to the tiny capillaries of the eye. The sweet fruit has been used for decades in Europe to treat vision problems ranging from night blindness to nearsightedness. In World War II, pilots in the Royal Air Force ate Bilberry jam to improve eyesight before night flights. Now, it's used to relieve eye strain from computer work and treat cataracts.

Besides improving vision, peripheral circulation and vascular health, Bilberry also acts as a mild diuretic. It stimulates the kidneys and combats diarrhea. Herbalist Maude Grieve recommends a tincture made from bruised roots steeped in gin to relieve edema.

Rich in beta carotene, vitamin E and flavanoids, the berries and leaves of the plant can be taken in tea, tincture or capsule. In Russia, the nutritious Bilberry is used to treat stomach conditions such as gastric colitis and to lower blood sugar in diabetics.

Bilberry is non-toxic. It is sold in capsules containing about 25 percent anthocyanosides, its active herbal constituent. Researchers have used dosages of up to 480 mg. per day without any adverse effects. Alone, Bilberry can be taken in a maintenance dose of 1-2 capsules per day, according to Mowrey. It can also be used in a tonic for the entire circulatory system.

Mowrey recommends a combination of Bilberry, Ginkgo, Gotu Kola and Ginger to strengthen and tone the blood vessels and capillaries in both peripheral and central circulation areas; support tissue repair by ensuring adequate blood flow to the affected areas and removal of toxins from the body; prevent free radical damage such as atherosclerosis and to forestall disorders of the central nervous system.

The suggested preventative dosage is 1-2 capsules a day. For treatment of acute and chronic conditions take 2-5 capsules per day.

Mowrey also recommends a combination of Bilberry, Gotu Kola, Butcher's Broom and Ginger root to prevent and treat circulatory disorders and build stronger blood vessels. By combining Bilberry and Butcher's Broom this formula might also help prevent aneurysms from forming. Mowrey recommends 1-2 capsules per day for prevention, 2-4 capsules for acute conditions and 1-4 capsules for chronic conditions.

Butcher's Broom (Latin name: *Ruscus Aculeatus*)

Recommended by Dioscorides, chief physician to the ancient Roman army, for the treatment of water retention caused by heart failure, Butcher's Broom has achieved prominence in Europe as a treatment for a variety of vascular disorders.

Butcher's Broom stimulates sluggish peripheral circulation, thins the blood and strengthens and tones fragile capillaries. It's one of the most commonly prescribed herbs for the treatment of such conditions as peripheral circulatory edema and phlebitis – inflammation of the veins due to insufficient circulation. Both are experienced by people with CHF.

In an experiment performed on rabbits, Butcher's Broom reduced the hyperpermeability or leakiness of diseased blood vessels in the animals and restored proper flow of nutrients and disposal of toxins. By targeting weak, leaky blood vessels, Butchers' Broom may be an effective treatment for aneurysm.

Incidentally, Butcher's Broom should not be confused with Broom (Sarothamnus Scoparius). The flowering tops of Broom can raise blood pressure and are toxic, while Butcher's Broom root is safe, nontoxic and does not raise blood pressure.

By increasing blood flow to the peripheral capillaries, Butcher's Broom also eases chilblains. Chilblains are an extreme sensitivity to cold resulting from insufficient circulation. While boosting blood flow to the affected tissues, the herb increases the elasticity of the capillary walls, strengthening the circulatory system.

While increasing circulation, French studies show Butcher's Broom decreases the likelihood of a surgical complication called thrombosis, where blood clots form in the blood stream and cause heart attack or stroke.

In a study spanning years and incorporating 1,654 patients, Dr. J.M. Verne found Butcher's Broom helped prevent postoperative thrombosis. Patients who were given the herb five days before a serious operation had a 1.8 percent chance of developing thrombosis. Without the herb, the incidence of thrombosis rose to 37.4 percent.

A part of herbal folklore for centuries, Butcher's Broom came into common usage after standardized forms were developed that offer reliable levels of ruscogenins, the active ingredient in the herb. Use guaranteed potency whole herb preparations to assure full medicinal value and safety.

Butcher's Broom is usually taken in tea or capsule form as part of a tonic for the prevention and treatment of vascular system disorders. A variety of circulatory blends with Butcher's Broom are now available. Mowrey recommends a mixture of Butcher's Broom, Ginger, Bilberry and Gotu Kola. (See Bilberry section for more information.) Butcher's Broom is non-toxic and has no side effects even in high doses.

DIURETICS

Dandelion (Latin name: *Taraxacum Officinale*)

A bane to cultivators of field and lawn, the Dandelion is a boon in herbal medicine. On sunny days, children blow the down off the wild weed to make wishes come true. For people with congestive heart failure, Dandelion makes a dream diuretic, replacing the potassium the process takes out.

Stimulating the kidneys to rid the body of excess water depletes vital minerals like potassium, shifting the electrolyte balance in the heart muscle. Potassium deficiency and the resulting electrolyte imbalance can aggravate

congestive heart failure by causing dangerous rhythm disturbances. Dandelion's high potassium content replenishes the
lost mineral and stabilizes the electrolyte balance.

Dandelion leaf has been compared for effectiveness to
the chemical diuretic Furosemide (brand name Lasix).
Dandelion root has been used to aid digestion and purify the
blood. Since both the root and leaf have medicinal properties of great benefit to people with congestive heart failure,
it may be best to mix them for maximum effect.

As a blood purifier, Dandelion root supports the kidney's
and liver's function of straining toxins from the blood
stream. It has been used since the 10th century to ease
edema, cure chronic liver congestion, soothe an irritable
gallbladder and treat rheumatism.

High in minerals such as calcium, phosphorus and iron,
Dandelion alkalizes the blood. Acidic blood, according to
prevailing German medical theory, causes heart disease and
triggers congestive heart failure. Acid blood circulating
through a failing heart worsens the damage, according to
Japanese research.

Recommended by some as a treatment for hypoglycemia and diabetes, Dandelion root has been shown to help
regulate blood sugar levels in experiments on animals.

Dandelion's effect on blood sugar may be due to its high
inulin content. Some researchers theorize that since inulin
has similar properties to insulin it may act as a temporary
substitute for insulin. Others attribute inulin's blood sugar-
regulating properties to its high fiber content and its
concentration of fructose which may even out blood sugar
fluctuations.

Dandelion can be drunk in tea or roasted-root coffee,
taken in capsules or drops, eaten as a salad or even sipped
as wine. The greens, which can be used in salads and sand-
wiches like lettuce or served boiled like spinach, are high in
vitamin A and contain more B_1, C and D than most
vegetables.

Safe even in high dosages, Dandelion root is contained in
many patent medicines for kidney and liver ailments and is
listed in the *U.S. Pharmacopoeia*. Tinctures are available containing both the leaf and root for maximum effect.

The recommended dosage of Dandelion tincture for
congestive heart failure is 1/2 to 1 teaspoon three times a

day starting early in the morning and ending late afternoon. Avoid taking Dandelion at night as the diuretic action might disturb much-needed sleep.

Hoffmann's tincture blend for the treatment of congestive heart failure mixes 1 part Dandelion leaf with 3 parts Hawthorn, 1 part Motherwort, 1 part Ginkgo, 1 part Linden Blossom and 1 part Cramp Bark. He recommends taking 1 teaspoonful three times a day.

Self-taught herbalist and author Dick Quinn concocted a very effective "water pill" containing 6 parts Dandelion leaf, 1 part Dandelion root, 6 parts Burdock root and one part Cayenne. He took the two "00" capsules once a day for maintenance and three times a day when edema appeared. Take the last capsules mid-afternoon so as not to disturb sleep.

A decoction can be made by boiling 2-3 teaspoons of the root in one pint of boiled water for 10 minutes and drunk three times a day. An infusion can be made by pouring boiling water over a cupful of Dandelion leaves. To make a medicinal tea containing both leaf and root, pour the hot Dandelion root decoction over the Dandelion leaves and steep 10-20 minutes.

Burdock (Latin name: *Arctium Lappa*)

Found along the roadside in the northern climates of Britain, the United States, Europe and Asia, Burdock is one of the best diuretics and blood purifiers nature has to offer.

Sporting button-shaped blue flowers, Burdock gets its botanical name from the Celtic word for "hand" because the burrs catch onto everything. It catches and disposes of toxins in the system three ways; as a diuretic, a diaphoretic and a blood purifier.

A diaphoretic, warm Burdock tea before a hot bath will "sweat out" toxins. Diaphoretic herbs open the pores of the skin for the volatile oils to "sweat out" toxins, renewing energy and generating a soothing warmth at the surface.

Burdock relieves edema by stimulating the kidneys, increasing the flow of urine. A demulcent, it also soothes the inflamed tissues of the bladder, kidney and liver. Edema from congestive heart failure puts an extra burden on the liver and kidneys that Burdock eases as it drains the excess fluid.

Cleansing the blood of toxins, Burdock boosts liver function. It works on the kidneys to de-acidify the blood and lower high blood sugar.

Burdock also has been used to reverse hardening of the arteries, treat inflammatory diseases such as rheumatism and clear skin disorders like eczema and psoriasis.

Since the diaphoretic properties are contained in the herb's volatile oils, Burdock root must not be boiled for tea, but rather steeped in a covered pot. The crushed seeds or powdered root can also be taken in capsule form. Fresh roots cut before the flowers open are very nutritious and taste like asparagus.

Burdock can be taken as a tincture, a tea, a decoction, a capsule or even eaten in a salad. For prevention, treatment and recovery, Burdock can be taken alone but is often combined with other herbs to bring its myriad benefits to those formulas. It mixes well with other diuretics such as Dandelion (See Quinn's diuretic formula in Dandelion section); cardiac tonics such as Cayenne, Hawthorn and Motherwort; or blood purifiers such as Sarsaparilla.

Herbalist Dr. John Christopher concocted a Burdock formula to purify the blood consisting of 4 tablespoons Burdock root, 4 tablespoons Yellow Dock, 1 tablespoon Blood Root and 1 pint of Glycerine. Simmer in $1\frac{1}{2}$ quarts boiling water until liquid has dropped by one-third. Sweeten with honey and glycerin (a preservative), bottle and store in cool place. The recommended dosage is one wine glass full 3-4 times a day.

If taken by itself, a decoction can be made from 1 teaspoon of the dried powdered root and drunk three times a day. The tincture dosage is 1-2 milliliters three times a day. The capsule dosage for reducing edema is 2 capsules three times daily, ending well before bedtime.

Cornsilk (Latin name: *Stigmata Maydis or Zea Mays*)

The fine, yellow threads covering kernels of Indian corn make one of the gentlest, most effective diuretics for congestive heart failure. As an anti-inflammatory herb, Cornsilk soothes the urinary system as it stimulates urine production and elimination.

Targeting edema caused by congestive heart failure, Cornsilk lowers blood pressure by reducing fluid retention. For that reason, it has been used in China for centuries to treat hypertension. It has also been used to regulate cholesterol and treat atherosclerosis.

Like the corn it wraps, Cornsilk is nutritious. Containing vitamins C and K, saponins and fatty acids, Cornsilk is one diuretic that nourishes rather than depletes the system, unlike many prescription diuretics.

Cornsilk can be found in many over-the-counter diuretics sold throughout Europe and the U.S. It can be taken alone or in combination with other herbal diuretics.

Mowrey recommends a diuretic blend of Cornsilk, Parsley, Uva-Ursi leaves, Buchu leaves, Cleavers, Juniper Berries, Kelp, Cayenne and Queen-of-the-Meadow Root. Mowrey's mixture is designed to relieve severe edema caused by congestive heart failure, purify the blood and nourish the body. For acute edema, take 5-8 capsules per day. In higher doses, Mowrey's diuretic formula can have the harmless side-effect of turning the urine a brownish color.

If taken alone, an infusion of Cornsilk can be made from two teaspoonfuls of the dried herb and drunk three times a day or taken as a tincture dosage of 2 milliliters three times a day. Capsule dosage for severe edema is 2 capsules three times a day, ending well before bedtime.

Parsley (Latin name: *Petroselinum Sativum*)

More commonly thought of for its culinary rather than curative properties, Parsley is one of the most nutritious diuretics.

The leafy green plant contains three times the amount of vitamin C as citrus juice and more iron than any other vegetable. High in vitamins A and B, Parsley juice has been used as a tonic for the blood vessels.

High levels of chlorophyll in Parsley make it a much-prescribed tonic for treating degenerative disease. Potassium contained in the aromatic herb helps replace the minerals lost in the diuretic process of draining excess water. As a nutritive herb, Parsley contains as much as 25 percent protein.

Used to treat everything from halitosis to high blood pressure, Parsley's ancient diuretic properties have been virtually ignored in modern times. Effective but gentle, Parsley soothes inflammation in the kidneys, liver and spleen. It also aids digestion, purifies the blood and boosts the immune system. As an antibacterial, it guards against infection.

A tonic for the entire body, Parsley regulates the adrenal glands, strengthens the sympathetic nervous system, tones the blood vessels and regulates blood pressure.

Parsley can be eaten by the sprig, taken in capsules or sipped in teas. It can be used alone or with other diuretics such as Cornsilk, Juniper Berry, Dandelion leaf and Burdock root.

Dr. Christopher recommends a blood circulation combination that blends Parsley with Ginger, Cayenne, Golden Seal, Ginseng and Garlic. The formula is designed to feed calcium to the circulatory system, stimulate circulation, cleanse the bloodstream, regulate blood pressure and restore elasticity to veins and blood vessels.

If taken by itself, an infusion made from 1-2 teaspoons of dried Parsley or a tincture dosage of 1-2 milliliters can be taken three times a day.

Juniper Berry (Latin name: *Juniperus Communis*)

Juniper Berry is a stimulating diuretic that targets kidney congestion resulting from congestive heart failure. It increases urine production, removes poisons from the bloodstream, enhances appetite and eases digestion.

Juniper Berry stimulates urine flow by increasing the rate at which the kidneys purify the blood and filter out wastes. An antiseptic as well as a diuretic, Juniper Berry helps heal the kidneys, bladder and urinary tract. It also dissolves kidney stones.

Besides soothing the urinary system, the dark purple berries have also been used to ease the pain of rheumatism and arthritis. As a bitter, the berries aid digestion and dispel flatulence.

Juniper Berry has been used to cleanse the system to ward off contagious illnesses by expelling the germs. As an expectorant, Juniper has been employed to treat colds and respiratory ailments.

Juniper Berry is usually part of a diuretic formula like Mowrey's which mixes Juniper Berry with Cornsilk, Parsley, Uva-Ursi, Cleavers, Buchu leaf, Kelp, Cayenne and Queen-of-the-Meadow root (See Cornsilk section). If taken alone, the dosage is 1 cupful of infusion or 1 milliliter of tincture three times a day.

While Juniper Berry – which is used to make gin and flavor foods – is nontoxic, it is not recommended for pregnant women or people with kidney disease due to its strong direct stimulation of the kidneys.

Elder (Latin name: *Sambucus Nigra*)

In ancient times, the Elder tree was used as a talisman against evil. In Sicily, travelers carried the sticks to protect themselves from snakes and thieves while the English cultivated it near their cottages to ward off witches. Congestive heart failure patients can use Elder to dispel edema.

Hippocrates, the Greek physician, employed almost the entire tree – bark, leaves, flowers and berries – as a diuretic and blood purifier. The root and leaves have been touted for centuries throughout Europe as one of the most effective treatments for the edema caused by congestive heart failure.

In old England, a charm made from the knotted twig was said to protect the body against rheumatism. Juice of Elder berries has been prescribed as a cure for rheumatism while a tea made from either the leaves or the dried berries is said to stop chronic diarrhea. The American Indians used an antiseptic liquid made from the flowers and leaves to treat skin conditions.

Hot Elderberry wine was sipped in the evenings to ward off a cold. Soup in Germany and syrup in Holland have been eaten to cleanse the system and stop fevers.

The medicinal characteristics of the Dwarf Elder (Sambucus Ebulus) are similar but more powerful than the common elder. Although there is little lore surrounding the smaller elder, Dwarf Elder leaves have been hailed as more effective in treatments for kidney and liver inflammation and cardiac edema.

The bark of its New England cousin, the American Dwarf Elder (Sambucus Canadensis) has also been used to treat edema and urinary problems while wine made from the berries is said to ease the pain of rheumatism. The berries themselves are rich in iron.

High in vitamin C, calcium and beta carotene, the Elder is a "spring cleaning" herb used to detoxify the body and throw off the colds and flu of winter. Taken with Peppermint, Elder helps "sweat out" colds, flu and respiratory ailments. As an expectorant, it's been used to relieve respiratory congestion.

Elder can be combined with other diuretic herbs to help fight edema and cleanse the blood or it can be taken on its own. An Elder infusion can be made using 2 tablespoons of the flowers and drunk three times a day. Tincture dosage (made of Elder flowers) is 2-4 milliliters three times a day.

Cleavers (Latin name: *Galium Aparine*)

A diuretic and one of the best tonics for the lymphatic system, Cleavers has been used to resolve a wide range of problems ranging from swollen glands to skin conditions and ulcers to edema.

By assisting the lymphatic system to drain properly, Cleavers helps detoxify the tissues. As an anti-inflammatory and antibiotic herb, it soothes irritation of the liver, kidneys and urinary tract and helps prevent infection.

Recent studies have also uncovered hypotensive properties in Cleavers. Used as a cleansing diuretic and glandular tonic in the treatment of the water retention and fatigue that come with congestive heart failure, Cleavers may also help regulate blood pressure which is both a cause and a symptom of CHF.

Cleavers is a complementary herb, usually taken as part of an herbal tonic. Mowrey's Diuretic Tonic combines Cleavers with Cornsilk, Parsley, Juniper Berries, Kelp, Cayenne, Buchu leaves and Queen-of-the-Meadow Root. He recommends 5-8 capsules be taken to treat acute edema.

If this blend is used, a potassium supplement should be considered. Dandelion leaf is one of the few diuretics that contain potassium to replace what is lost when excess water is drained from the body.

An infusion of Cleavers can be made from 2 teaspoons of dried herb and taken three times a day. Tincture dosage is 2-4 milliliters three times a day.

FINDING AN HERBALIST

The healing plants discussed in this chapter are only part of what herbalism has to offer in the fight against congestive heart failure. There are no stronger advocates for the prevention of illness, and the individualistic approach herbalists take to treatment encompasses the whole person – mind, body and soul.

As much an intuitive art as a holistic science, herbalism looks at each individual and tries to ascertain what interfered with their body's natural defenses and healing mechanisms. Herbalists probe deep into the patient's family history, diet, lifestyle, frustrations, hopes and dreams to identify the causes of conditions like congestive heart failure.

"From an herbalist's perspective, giving cardioactive medication doesn't address the underlying cause," said Upton, president of the American Herbalists Guild. "Why do they have high blood pressure? Is it stress, fluid retention, thick blood?

"We start by dealing with the underlying cause and manifestation of the condition with diet, lifestyle and stress reduction. We don't just give them a magic bullet," he said.

The herbalist's goal is to help patients heal themselves by putting them back in touch with their own bodies. If the approach of allopathic (drug-based) medicine can be compared to the way an auto mechanic fixes a broken down car, the herbalist mechanic gives the customer the tools to do regular tune-ups themselves to keep the car running smoothly and avoid future breakdowns.

"Herbs give the body what it needs (to heal)," explained herbalist James Green, author of *The Male Herbal*. "Its natural condition is bliss and health – it's always looking for a balance with its own unique nature. Give it the tools it needs and then give it time."

Herbalism educates the patient so they understand how to regain their health and keep it. "It's the same as with most natural healing modalities because let's face it, you come to see a practitioner once a week or once a month and then the rest of the time you're on your own," Upton said. "You should be living in a way that takes care of yourself."

Empowering patients to be responsible for their own health makes sense, Upton said, since there are some elements in their recovery only they can control such as their mental health and emotional well-being.

Herbalists strive to impart the kind of "health" embodied in the World Health Organization's definition of the term: "Health is more than simply the absence of illness. It is the active state of physical, emotional, mental and social well-being."

To help the patient achieve full health, herbalists embrace the patient's individuality rather than trying to fit them into a standard patient profile. This personalized, all-encompassing approach to healing can have remarkable effects in the prevention and early treatment of serious conditions like congestive heart failure.

"Herbs are used for prevention first," Green said. "Next, for treating minor ailments and then for nourishing, toning and rebuilding the body to get rid of chronic ailments. But when you get to a crisis, you look at intervention and that's where allopathic medicine comes in – crisis intervention. You use herbal tonics to support that."

Severe congestive heart failure is one example of a serious illness that benefits greatly by combining the best natural and allopathic medicine have to offer. Crisis medicines pull the patient back from the brink and treat the symptoms of CHF while herbal cardiac tonics rebuild strength, reactivate the body's own healing mechanisms and uncover the cause to stop further damage.

"Herbalism is not an alternative to allopathic medicine – it's complementary," Green explained. "It's a holistic approach to healing."

Unfortunately, this holistic approach to health care has not been wholly accepted by either the American medical establishment or the legislators.

Herbalists in this country are relegated to a supporting role. Currently, herbalists have no legal right to operate as primary care physicians while herb-trained naturopathic doctors, acupuncturists and practitioners of Traditional Chinese Medicine (TCM) are allowed to diagnose and treat patients.

"Herbalists by themselves are not legal to practice without an acupuncturist or naturopathic physician's license," Upton explained. "Ordinary people have the right to use herbs, but that's not the same as prescribing herbs for treatment."

Most of the 500 members of the American Herbalists Guild are licensed and those who are not are teachers, Upton said. While there is no official regulatory body for herbalists, the American Herbalists Guild accepts and certifies its membership based on peer review.

Prospective members must have at least three years of experience, three references from professional herbalists, documented education and training, and a completed questionnaire testing the depth of their knowledge and experience. The applicants' materials are reviewed by a peer panel made up of five herbalist from various orientations. Approval must be unanimous to earn the title Herbalist, AHG.

Practitioners of traditional Chinese medicine, acupuncture or naturopathic medicine learn about herbal medicine as part of their training. Herbalists specialize in the use of the green medicines and the philosophy surrounding them.

The herbal practitioner's approach varies depending on the type of training they have received. Naturopathic doctors (N.D.) use diagnostic techniques that mirror those of medical doctors (M.D.) since their training is similar. However, naturopathic doctors use non-invasive therapies to treat the patient including homeopathic medicines, nutritional supplements, dietary regimens, stress reduction and other lifestyle changes.

Practitioners of Traditional Chinese Medicine (TCM) include licensed acupuncturists (L.Ac.), oriental medical doctors (O.M.D.) and independent oriental herbalists working under a Diplomat of Chinese Herbology certificate granted by the National Commission for Certification of Acupuncturists (NCCA). TCM practitioners have their own unique brand of diagnostic techniques and treatment therapies.

In China, doctors commonly treat heart disease using a five-step approach that begins with lifestyle modification, stress reduction and exercises like Tai Chi, according to Upton. The second step is the use of herbal formulas tailored to the particular needs of the patient, followed by pharmaceutical and herbal diuretics. Conventional medicines such as beta blockers and hypertensive drugs don't even enter the picture until the fourth stage. Surgical intervention is the fifth and last resort.

According to Upton's research, more than two-thirds of these heart patients can be successfully treated using the first three steps while most of the patients who've reached the fourth stage can avoid the need for surgery using the non-invasive methods.

Since the United States has yet to recognize the contribution of herbalists as medical practitioners, they often serve as an adjunct to a primary allopathic physician. In that role, the herbalist's recommendations are based on the physician's diagnosis. Even so, the herbalist often offers a deeper evaluation of the causes of the condition.

A competent herbalist can design an herbal treatment program that will target the causes of the congestive heart failure and support the conventional allopathic treatment by maximizing the effectiveness of such medications as Digitalis, nourishing the circulatory system and easing edema without depleting critical potassium levels.

Herbal practitioners can also guide patients seeking to wean themselves off certain drugs by helping correct the problem the drugs are prescribed to treat or offering safe herbal alternatives. Powerful cardiac herbs like Lily of the Valley and Cactus Grandiflorus are best used under the care of an herbal practitioner – especially if the goal is to substitute the herbs for the drug Digitalis. This can be a dangerous undertaking for patients with severe congestive heart failure and should only be attempted under medical supervision.

Since they operate in a legal "gray area" and are not protected by any regulatory body, Herbalists safeguard themselves and their patients with "Informed Consent." Informed Consent is a health contract of sorts detailing the herbalist's background, training and experience; the proposed treatment plan; the costs and the expectations of both parties.

As a practicing herbalist for seven years, Upton authored his own Informed Consent contracts which outlined realistic expectations and emphasized that the patient must share in the responsibility of restoring their health.

"I stressed four points: This is the best information I can give you; this should be done in conjunction with a licensed physician; I have no idea how it's really going to work for you because everyone is different; and that most of work to be done is within your lifestyle," Upton explained. "And that's the reality of health care. It's not just a way of legally covering your butt!"

In recent years, a growing number of allopathic doctors have begun to tap into the many benefits natural medicine has to offer their patients. Those medical doctors who can get past prejudice against "alternative medicine" are reaching out to natural practitioners and pulling them closer to the mainstream.

As their popularity grows, herbalists like Green are concerned about being submerged in a conventional approach to medicine they support but do not espouse.

"We need to maintain our own identity, not just become another part of allopathic medicine," Green said. "We are complementary but different. If it becomes just another bottle on the shelf – a "green" allopathic medicine – then we've lost our connection to the earth.

"These are medicines you can make in your home, cook in your kitchen and use to attend to minor ailments and nourish yourself," he said. "What we really need to do is change the definition of mainstream medicine and put the emphasis on nourishing the body and preventing disease. Nothing else makes sense."

The American Herbalists Guild can help you find a qualified herbalist in your area. For the membership directory, send $2 to: The American Herbalists Guild, P.O. Box 746555, Arvada, CO 80006 or call (303) 423-8800.

To locate a naturopath, contact the American Association of Naturopathic Physicians (AANP) at (206) 323-7610 or send a $5 referral list fee to AANP, 2366 East Lake Ave. E., Seattle, WA 98102.

A practitioner of Traditional Chinese Medicine or Acupuncture can be found through the American Association of Oriental Medicine (AAOM), 433 Front St., Catasauqua, PA 18032-2526. The association, which provides free referrals to over 1,200 members who hold both a national certification and a state license, can also be reached by calling (610) 266-1433.

Licensed health care practitioners who also have homeopathic training are listed by the National Center for Homeopathy, 801 North Fairfax Street, Suite 306, Alexandria, VA 22314. For the directory of over 400 members, send $6 or call (703) 548-7790.

The Holistic Health Directory and Resource Guide offers a comprehensive list of over 7,000 practitioners of 100 categories of alternative therapies. The directory is available at health stores and book stores for $5.95.

Information on these and other referral agencies, research centers and treatment methods is available through the American Holistic Association. The non-profit volunteer agency can be reached by calling (714) 779-6152 or write to P.O. Box 17400 Anaheim, CA 92817.

For more information on herbs and alternative medicine contact:

The Herb Research Foundation
1007 Pearl Street Ste. 200
Boulder, CO. 80302
(303) 449-2265

World Research Foundation
15300 Ventura Blvd. Ste. 405
Sherman Oaks, CA 91403
(818) 907-5483

SECTION IV

FUELING THE FIGHT AGAINST HEART FAILURE

If I'd known I would live this long,
I would have taken better care of myself.

-ANONYMOUS

PART ONE: FOOD CHOICES AND HEART FAILURE

Dick Quinn always referred to me as "My friend Al Watson." We met at a hospital in 1982. He was a writer selling "business mail," and I was a "public relations assistant manager." Our department was doing a neighborhood mailing to attract new patients. As fate would have it, Dick had sent the hospital his "You and I have something in common" letter. We were favorably impressed – just the guy to spice up our direct mail efforts.

I was assigned to work with Dick. During our initial meeting, I noticed Dick popping red capsules. I had to ask.

He didn't hesitate to tell me. Double-bypass surgery that didn't work; "The lady at the lake" who had introduced him to Cayenne pepper; and finally, Cayenne to the rescue. The same story would be heard on hundreds of radio stations 10 years later.

As it turned out, "Quinn" and I had a lot in common. We drove old American cars (he drove only convertibles). For a time, we were network news junkies. We got together just to watch taped news programs, loudly discussing world problems. Each December, we made our pilgrimage to Dick's farm to cut down a couple of Christmas trees. And I, too, had lost my father at the age of nine. Although we botched the hospital mailing (the response was less than 1 percent), Quinn and I became close friends.

Summer, 1989: Dick and I were excited about our new businesses. He had lost interest in his direct mail agency, and I had long since been asked to leave St. John's Hospital. He was going to start selling his Cayenne formulas and I wanted to open an herb store.

By December, Quinn was making capsules in the living room of his apartment. I was his first customer – selling "Power Caps" in a new herb store with the unlikely name, "Earth Chicken."

The Earth Chicken – let's just say – was ahead of its time. After a few years, it went gracefully out of business. Dick offered me a position at Heart Foods which was now operating out of an abandoned supermarket in one of the toughest neighborhoods in Minneapolis.

I was in charge the day the Food & Drug Administration (FDA) came through the front door and ordered our best customer to stop selling our products in its catalog. The FDA objected to a "claim" in our advertising that suggested Cayenne was good for the heart.

Down on our luck, we moved the company to an abandoned liquor store owned by the city of Minneapolis. Here we continued production and started searching for a permanent home. There were missed paydays, but mail order sales were sustaining the company during its darkest hour. While I was "running" Heart Foods, Dick was busy writing *Left For Dead*. It was early 1992.

Left For Dead saved Heart Foods. Sales were taking off

again. More importantly, *Left For Dead* was a triumph for Dick – fulfilling a dream. In March 1992, Dick severed all ties with Heart Foods and started the R.F. Quinn Publishing Company.

In March, 1993, he moved to San Clemente, California, to be close to his two daughters. I was the only other officer of R.F. Quinn Publishing and its General Manager. Dick was on the move – the star of the 1993 "Left For Dead Tour."

By early 1994, however, something was wrong with Dick Quinn. I met Dick at the Wyndham Hotel in New York City around midnight on March 14. He arrived from Florida completely exhausted.

At 1 am, Dick suggested we go out and get a bite to eat. We walked a couple of blocks to a 24-hour deli. Dick had to walk slowly, feeling constant pain in his lower back and groin.

As he enjoyed his cheeseburger, French fries and coffee with sugar and half-and-half, he explained how he'd had a "scary experience" a few weeks earlier in a Texas hotel room. He experienced sudden, crushing fatigue and shortness of breath.

The episode passed, but his energy and stamina were never the same after that, he said. In Florida, a nutritionist had set him up with a wide array of vitamin and mineral supplements – adding a few more pounds to his heavy luggage.

He and the luggage he carried around were both gaining weight. (Dick was an inveterate book buyer.) He was agitated about his pending divorce from his second wife, Paula, and he feared that he could lose part of R.F. Quinn Publishing. After a talk and book-signing at Willner Chemists in New York City, we were off by rental car to a nutritional foods conference in Montreal.

It was March 17, 1994 – St. Patrick's Day. Always a special day for Quinn, this was the day of his second divorce (he participated by telephone) which he celebrated that evening at an Irish pub. At the conference we attended that day, he had appeared overweight, sweaty and tired. He insisted on taking cabs short distances. He talked incessantly about problems with his California office, the divorce and his rigid schedule.

Throughout '93 and '94, it was go-go-go for Dick

Quinn. Not much rest and relaxation. Very few walks on the beach in beautiful San Clemente. Like a lot of people, Dick was driven.

In business and life, he moved along in the fast lane. He could be very impatient at times. He once told me, "Al, I'm a poor waiter – I hate to wait for anything." He was stressed when things didn't go as planned. Even then, he would take on more projects and responsibilities.

New Year's Eve, 1994: I arrived in San Clemente around 11 p.m. Two weeks earlier, Dick had been given 24-hours to live. He had been diagnosed with heart failure. His bulging aortic aneurysm had not been detected yet.

When I arrived at 410 Victoria Street, Dick was sleeping in his chair, carnation in his coat, newspapers scattered about. Despite his apparent weakness, he insisted we go to "Tommy's" for a bite to eat.

Like New York City nine months earlier, it was 1 a.m. and Dick Quinn was eating a cheeseburger, French fries and coffee with sugar and half-and-half. Though I knew this couldn't be good for him – salting every single bite – I also sensed that he was enjoying his food and didn't need a lecture from me.

We knew each other well. He didn't want to be "hard-assed" about nutrition, especially on New Year's Eve. Back home at his apartment, he insisted that we have dessert – his favorite – coconut cake and ice cream.

St. Patrick's Day, 1995: Three months later, I'm back in San Clemente. Dick had nearly died again. His heart function had declined dramatically and he was on oxygen.

He was very weak but he wanted to celebrate St. Patrick's Day with a Guinness. Getting dressed, walking down to the car and unloading at the bar were too much for Quinn. Although we managed to reach a seat, without ordering, we made the slow, painful trip back to Dick's apartment.

Dick had always said, "I can eat what I want and not worry about it." Not anymore. A sip of beer or a bite of dessert could bring on prolonged stomach pain and indigestion.

Plagued with water buildup (edema), shortness of breath and staggering fatigue, Dick had a lot to worry about.

Seventeen years after bouncing back from failed coronary bypass surgery, Dick had learned that Cayenne was not a total therapy for heart disease.

In 1978, it was Cayenne to the rescue. Six months after his bypass, his coronary arteries had clamped down. The fiery, quick stimulant action of Cayenne dramatically improved blood volume to his heart.

Cayenne brought Dick back from the dead in 1978. His wife Elaine and five children saw it with their own eyes. In his dying months of 1995, however, there was no botanical equivalent – no "magic bullet" for his failing heart.

Dick had become a seat-of-the-pants herbalist. He knew a lot about herbs – especially Cayenne. Like any therapy, herbs are more effective with a balanced natural foods diet.

Quinn referred to himself as "Mr. Cheeseburger," a self-described nutritionist's nightmare. And he was. Dietary excesses were a part of him. Plenty of feed-lot meat, bacon, eggs and cheeseburgers. Salt on everything. He seldom prepared salads or vegetables. Even after he was stricken with heart failure, he continued eating sweet rolls, donuts and big bowls of coconut cake and ice cream.

A donut once in a while won't kill you. Eggs from free-range chickens, one or two a day, are good for most people. High-quality red meat can restore vitality in weak persons. But eating excessive amounts of any food – even good foods – may kill you.

Dick ate too much red meat at the expense of vegetables. He fried eggs in poor-quality cooking oils. He often ate a steak sandwich late at night, just before going to bed. He slept late. Breakfast out often included eggs, bacon or sausage, pancakes and a donut. He drank coffee or iced tea (with sugar and half-and-half) throughout the day.

Mel Boyd, a friend of Dick's in Minneapolis, saw it coming as early as 1989. He feared that Dick was over-stimulating himself with Cayenne, red meat and sugar. When he suggested moderation one day at a business lunch, Dick laughed him off.

In a sense, Dick was the quintessential American reaching maturity in the '50s. He didn't think anyone, including himself, should be troubled with biochemistry. Besides, eating was a lot of fun – fuel for the great American hustle to get ahead.

To Dick, Cayenne was a magic shield protecting him against his most feared enemy – a heart attack. Dick accomplished that, but he failed to take the next and most important step: balancing his diet with a variety of wholesome natural foods.

Considering that all four of his grandparents and both parents died relatively young of circulatory disorders, it would have made sense for Dick, who suffered a major heart attack at the age of 42, to take dietary and nutritional issues more seriously. Because he didn't, at age 58, he found himself up against an even more confounding enemy: late-stage congestive heart failure.

PART TWO: PATHWAYS TO HEART FAILURE

Congestive heart failure doesn't have a single cause – just as it doesn't have a single solution. Hereditary and congenital factors, dietary imbalances and nutritional deficiencies all underlie its development.

Elevated blood pressure is the most common early warning that the heart and vascular network are in a state of "dis-ease." (Dick Quinn's high blood pressure had distended his aorta by age 42.) Lack of exercise, stress and unresolved emotional problems all contribute to heart disease, heart attack and heart failure.

Food choices can either protect us from heart failure or promote vascular breakdown. There's a lot of truth in the old family doctor's admonition to "eat a balanced diet" for good health. There's a lot of disagreement, though, about just what that means.

Conflicting dietary advice and misinformation has reached epidemic proportions. Too often nutritional information is provided by commercial interests and government agencies under their influence.

In 1985, the National Cholesterol Education Program officially launched its "War on cholesterol."

Interest in cholesterol as a heart disease risk factor grew out of the long-term Framingham Population Study (Framingham is a city in Massachusetts) begun in 1948. Researchers found a modest correlation between high serum (blood) cholesterol and incidence of heart disease in young and middle-age men and, to a lesser degree, in women between the ages of 40-50.

This correlation between high blood cholesterol and increased risk of coronary artery disease declined in both men and women at about age 50 and then disappeared entirely. Among the elderly, the group in which most deaths from coronary artery disease occur, high blood cholesterol levels did not appear to be a risk factor. The Framingham data also showed extensive heart disease among people with low or average blood cholesterol.

The war on cholesterol went public largely on the basis of this inconclusive Framingham data and two even less convincing government-sponsored studies costing $494 million – MR. FIT and the Coronary Primary Prevention Trial (CPPT).

A massive advertising program was launched with millions of dollars from the federal government, the American Medical Association, the pharmaceutical industry and cereal manufacturers. Without anything resembling scientific proof, a "consensus conference" of doctors and government bureaucrats decided that dietary cholesterol from animal products determined blood cholesterol levels and that this elevated blood cholesterol was the primary cause of coronary artery disease.

Inaccurate testing methods, low-cholesterol diets that had not been clinically evaluated and expensive new anti-cholesterol drugs were approved in record time. Americans by the millions marched back and forth to their doctors to get their cholesterol checked. We dutifully switched from butter to newly labeled "heart smart" margarine. Oils that never contained animal products were marketed as "cholesterol free." Once known as the "perfect food," eggs became cholesterol booby traps. We switched to egg-whites and Egg-beaters®.

Yet most of us left the doctor's office with little to show for our participation in the government's final assault on heart disease. Our cholesterol numbers didn't budge and even went up. Low-cholesterol diets were not reducing cho-lesterol or the incidence of coronary artery disease – just as they had failed to do in either MR. FIT or the CPPT.

Studies in both Europe and the U.S. showed that people taking anti-cholesterol drugs had increased mortality from cancer, gallstones, accidents and suicide – canceling any possible benefit of taking the drug to reduce the chance of heart disease.

Today, we are learning the truth. There was and is no scientific evidence that high blood cholesterol is the cause of heart disease or that lowering cholesterol with diet – if it's even possible – will help you live longer.

Many things influence blood cholesterol. Eating dam-aged fats like margarine can increase blood cholesterol. Prescription drugs, such as high blood pressure medica-tions routinely given to heart patients, can increase blood cholesterol. High insulin levels and other disruptions of normal body chemistry also contribute to elevated blood cholesterol.

Cholesterol compounds are essential for life and are found in practically every cell of the body. Cholesterol lines our arteries, providing a slick surface for coursing blood. When a lesion develops on an arterial wall, cholesterol com-pounds are used to soothe and heal the injury. Like a high fever when a virus attacks, elevated cholesterol can be seen as the body's defensive response to arterial injury.

Cholesterol is carried in the blood to arteries and tissues in a fat-protein molecule called Low Density Lipoprotein (LDL). Excess cholesterol is carried away from the tissues back to the liver for disposal in a fat-protein vehicle called High Density Lipoprotein (HDL). Contrary to popular belief, LDL is not strictly "bad" and HDL is not "good."

Without LDL transport vehicles, cholesterol would not reach its destination. Referring to LDL as "bad" cholesterol is like calling emergency vehicles at the scene of an accident "bad." Chronically elevated LDL like is the body sending out a fleet of emergency vehicles to one of those chain-reac-tion freeway accidents involving dozens of cars. It's the acci-dent that's bad – not the presence of emergency vehicles.

Relatively high HDL levels in the blood (as a percentage of LDL) indicate that, biochemically, all is well. HDL mole-cules are like the city trucks hauling glass, paper and aluminum cans. They are not "good," they are simply doing their job, hauling vital materials – fats and cholesterol – back to the liver for recycling.

The only "bad" cholesterol is cholesterol that has been removed from circulation because it was "highjacked" by free radicals – the highly reactive chemical compounds created by radiation, environmental toxins, heat and chemical processing of foods, and normal body metabolism. Oxidized cholesterol represents the emergency vehicles piling up against each other and being damaged in the process.

The liver manufactures between one and four grams per day of cholesterol for circulation in the blood (an egg, in comparison, contains about one-quarter of a gram). Studies have shown that reductions or increases of dietary cholesterol have little, if any, bearing on blood cholesterol levels.

According to Thomas J. Moore, author of *Heart Failure*, volunteers (prisoners and students) eating up to 12 eggs a day for extended periods of time did not increase their serum cholesterol significantly. Like blood pressure, the body sets a cholesterol level for itself based on a wide range of biochemical and metabolic events that are not completely understood.

Meanwhile, there's not much evidence that Americans are benefiting from the assault on cholesterol. In 1989, heart disease killed more than 750,000 people. Heart failure represents the largest Medicare expenditure. The January 16, 1995 issue of *Time* magazine reports, "Despite the health craze, Americans are fatter than ever."

While fat consumption fell in the last decade, the percentage of overweight Americans increased. Today, at least one out of every four adults is 20 percent or more over ideal body weight.

Americans are the fattest people on earth. And it's not just a vanity issue. Weight gain is associated with high blood pressure, high insulin levels, diabetes and heart disease.

Our Modern Food Supply

Among various cultures around the world, people eating "whole" food diets made up of fresh, unprocessed grains, beans, vegetables and varying amounts of meat, dairy and fruit remain free of the degenerative diseases common in the United States today.

These heart-protective diets always consist of hearty, nutritious staple foods like brown rice, corn and rye. They never include damaged fats, refined carbohydrates and the convenience foods Americans consume in large quantities.

Healthy traditional diets may be high in fat. High fat diets are heart-protective when they are part of a natural foods diet suited to the climate, culture and metabolic needs of the people. For example, although 70 percent of their calories come from the fat of fish and other marine animals, Eskimos on a traditional diet do not get clogged arteries.

The high-fat diet of pioneer America was also a high-fiber diet. Bread was coarse, dark and nutritious. Crude vegetable oils contained vitamin E and lecithin. Meat was wild or range fed. Foraging chickens knew best. Soups were thick with vegetables grown in mineral-rich soil. The fiber of rye, wheat, oats and vegetables helped promote digestion, regular bowel movements and sound intestinal health – all mandatory in a high-saturated fat diet.

What has changed in America since 1910 is not our consumption of much vilified saturated fat, but the dramatic reduction in the fiber and nutritional content of staple foods. Chemical fertilizers and other modern farming practices have led to a decline in the quality of our meat, eggs and vegetables. This degradation of our food supply inversely parallels the steady increase in heart disease after 1910.

Today, the standard American diet (SAD) is not our diet of 1910. In part, heart and vascular diseases which lead to heart failure are a consequence of modern food processing. Staple foods like potatoes have become frozen French fries. Whole grains have become frosted-flakes. Coarse, dark bread has become white and light. The commercial processing of vegetable oils gained shelf life at the expense of nutritional value. Sweeteners, colors and preservatives have replaced fiber and nutrition in thousands of convenience foods.

The milling of whole wheat into "enriched" white flour began in the 1890s. Whole wheat was stripped of its germ and bran and chemicals were added to produce a free-flowing flour. "Enriching" white flour with three synthetic vitamins (B_1, B_2, B_3) and iron does not make up for the fiber and more than 30 other beneficial nutrients lost in the milling process.

Enriched white bread contains 90 percent less vitamin E, 80 percent less vitamin B_6 and 70 percent less magnesium and chromium than whole grain bread. Processing whole grains into white bread, white rice, white crackers, white noodles, dry cereals, pancakes, cookies and pastries has done more than remove nutritional value. Along with the vitamins and minerals went most of the fiber.

Fiber is what makes foods "whole." Though fiber itself has no nutritional value, fiber provides "nutritional effect." The fiber in fruits, vegetables and whole grains delays the entry of glucose into the bloodstream, helping to stabilize blood sugar levels.

Fiber also reduces the level of fats (triglycerides) circulating in the blood. Fiber is needed in the 20-foot long gastrointestinal tract to provide a buffer against toxins and to help eliminate waste materials. Fiber speeds up the transit time of body wastes and promotes detoxification.

Disturbed Carbohydrate Metabolism

In his new book *Enter The Zone*, based on Nobel Prize-winning research, Barry Sears, Ph.D. names high insulin levels – not cholesterol – as the best predictor of heart disease. While high blood cholesterol is modestly associated with heart disease in adults under age 50, high insulin levels are a major pathway to heart failure for everyone.

A biochemist and researcher, Sears blames popular low-fat, high-carbohydrate diets for driving up insulin levels and promoting heart disease. Sears cites Stanford University research indicating that approximately 25 percent of the U.S. population (about 60 million people) respond to excess dietary carbohydrates – even complex carbohydrates – by producing too much insulin.

Insulin is a hormone that regulates glucose (blood sugar), the body's basic energy fuel. If you eat a lot of carbohydrates, you'll produce a lot of glucose.

Insulin metabolizes glucose, converting it to immediate energy or storing it as fat. Insulin stores excess glucose as a fatty tissue called triglyceride – better known as body fat.

The rate at which carbohydrates enter the bloodstream is known as the "glycemic index." The lower the index, the slower the rate of glucose entry into the bloodstream. Slower entry of glucose into the bloodstream means more stable blood sugar levels.

Because the sugar in fruit must first be converted by the liver into glucose, fruits are low on the glycemic index. Because pasta, bread and grains contain glucose, they are high on the index and enter the bloodstream fastest.

The higher the fiber content of a carbohydrate, the lower it is on the glycemic index. Fiber-rich natural foods produce steady blood sugar levels. Highly-refined carbohydrates accelerate the rate of glucose entry. When glucose enters the bloodstream too fast, the pancreas responds by secreting high levels of insulin – in at least 25 percent of the population.

This overproduction of insulin in genetically sensitive individuals creates unstable blood sugar levels and encourages fat storage. According to Sears, this extremely powerful hormonal action promotes heart disease by increasing the tendency of blood to form unwanted clots and by constricting the arteries, increasing blood pressure.

What about the rest of us who are not genetically programmed to overproduce insulin? We set in motion the same hormonal chain of events by eating excess quantities of refined carbohydrates, those fiber-removed denatured foods that release glucose into our systems too quickly.

Because consumption of highly refined carbohydrates and sugar has grown steadily in the U.S. throughout the century, today as many as 100 million people may be susceptible to glucose-insulin disorders.

"Entering The Zone," says Sears, is the key to stable blood sugar levels. Stable blood sugar levels help prevent obesity, diabetes and heart disease. People in the "Zone" maintain steady blood sugar levels and hormonal balance with the proper mix of protein, carbohydrates and natural fats in each meal. Sears has defined scientifically what the old family doctor has been telling us for years: "Eat a balanced diet."

Protein foods balance carbohydrate-induced insulin by producing the hormone "glucagon." Glucagon acts as a brake on the release of insulin. While insulin metabolizes glucose, drives down blood sugar and locks up fat; protein-induced glucagon increases blood sugar and mobilizes fats from storage tissue.

The balance of insulin and glucagon depends on moderate-sized meals and a proper ratio of protein to carbohydrates in the diet. Consuming 2-4 ounces of high quality protein in each meal helps maintain stable blood sugar levels by the action of the insulin-glucagon balance.

Carbohydrates and proteins share a hormonal teeter-totter. If carbohydrate is too heavy, insulin shoots up. If carbohydrate and protein foods are in balance, the teeter-totter is more steady – no one gets hurt. Metabolic stability promotes hormonal stability, which promotes healthy body functioning.

In the same sense, yo-yo dieting upsets hormonal balance. Constantly shifting weight – up and down – will increase arterial plaque. A balanced diet is the key.

Like protein, dietary fats also slow the entry of carbohydrates into the bloodstream. Butter or natural peanut butter on bread will slow the release of glucose contained in the bread. Although protein foods contain fat, extra sources of unprocessed fat (the equivalent of one tablespoon) should be included in each meal.

By adding protein and healthy natural fat to each meal, stable blood sugar levels can be achieved. Healthy fats include unprocessed vegetable oils like safflower oil, flax seed oil, borage oil, virgin olive oil, avocados, nuts (in the shell) and seeds (raw or home roasted). Dietary fats add taste to food and their slow digestion helps promote a feeling of fullness.

If you are overweight or gain weight easily, you may be one of the 60 million Americans overproducing insulin after eating carbohydrates. Sugar cravings and hunger, weakness, irritability, headaches or moodiness within three hours of eating point to unstable blood sugar levels or hypoglycemia (low blood sugar).

If you have these symptoms after a carbohydrate meal or snack, you need to balance your meals with additional protein and natural fat. If you subsequently notice that your energy levels become more stable, it's because your blood sugar levels are more stable.

Whether or not you are genetically programmed to overproduce insulin, you can remove symptoms of hypoglycemia by removing all sugars, refined flours and processed foods from your diet. Emphasize whole, unrefined high-fiber foods low on the glycemic index like lentils, peas and beans instead.

Robert Atkins, MD, author of *Dr. Atkins' New Diet Revolution*, recommends that people with a family history of heart disease and 15 pounds to lose ask their doctor for a glucose tolerance test (usually covered by insurance). For the test, a large dose of glucose is given on an empty stomach and blood is drawn every hour over a four to five hour period to help identify blood sugar disorders.

People with blood sugar instability and those in search of optimum health may want to calculate their precise daily protein requirement. In *Enter The Zone*, Sears offers a personalized survey that calculates protein requirements based on weight, percentage of body fat and level of physical activity.

Dr. Atkins' New Diet Revolution also provides a way to arrive at your personal carbohydrate-protein mix and includes recipes to balance each meal.

Refined Sweeteners

Sugar is a highly processed product. Chemically similar to cocaine, sugar has no nutritional value. Not a large part of the traditional American diet, refined sweeteners like white sugar became popular in the 1890s after Coca Cola was introduced. Since then, sugar in our diet has become a vicious circle. As many of us know, eating sugar makes you want more sugar.

Sugar is a metabolic "freeloader," robbing your body of essential nutrients. Sugar interferes with the transport of vitamin C, depletes B-vitamins and blocks the absorption of minerals. Sugar stimulates the liver to produce more cholesterol. Excess sugar – and it doesn't take much – upsets blood sugar levels and hormonal balance.

Like other high glycemic-index carbohydrates, sugar consumption is linked to the overproduction of insulin, hypoglycemia, fatigue, weight gain, diabetes and heart disease.

According to Ann Louise Gittleman MS., author of *Beyond Pritikin*, in the last 20 years, the per capita ingestion of sugar has increased dramatically. Today, Americans are consuming over 130 pounds per person per year, hidden, to a large degree, in soft drinks, convenience foods, cookies, ice cream, salad dressings, sauces, ready-to-eat cereals and literally thousands of packaged food items on supermarket shelves.

The vast majority of the ready-to-eat commercial breakfast cereals derive 20 percent or more of their calories from sugar. For example, Nabisco Raisin Bran is 42 percent sugar. General Mills Cocoa Puffs are 47 percent sugar. Kellogg's Frosted Flakes are 43 percent sugar. Healthy-sounding cereals like Multi-grain Cheerios, All-Bran, and Quaker 100% Natural cereal are 20 percent or more sugar.

The combination of refined sugar and refined grains puts these cereals at the top of the glycemic index – sure to spike up insulin levels. When consumed with homogenized whole or 2% milk, you are adding damaged, potentially dangerous fat to your breakfast as well.

The Fate of Fats

Natural dietary fats supply the building blocks for the body's hormone production and are the main constituent of all cell membranes. Fatty structures are the body's chief defense against toxins. Throughout the body, fat acts as the "good cop," insulating and cushioning cells, tissues and organs while protecting them from invading toxins.

All fats, saturated (from meat) and unsaturated (from vegetables and fish), are efficient sources of energy for the body, but some fats are "essential."

Essential fatty acids are unsaturated fats that cannot be made in the body and must be provided in our diet. There are two essential fatty acids: Omega-3 alpha-linolenic acid and Omega-6 linoleic acid.

The Omega-3 and Omega-6 fatty acids are converted by the body into short-lived hormones called "prostaglandins." Made by every cell in the body, prostaglandins control every vital physiological function including the thickness of our blood and the flexibility of our arteries. Without these essential fats, hormone balance is not possible.

Dietary sources of Omega-3 include flax oil, cold-water fatty fish (salmon is best), and wild game. Flax oil is the richest plant source of Omega-3 (alpha-linolenic acid). In a healthy body, alpha-linolenic acid is converted into eicosapentaenoic acid (EPA).

EPA, in turn, is used by the body to build the beneficial prostaglandins that reduce blood fats, dissolve hard fats in the body and prevent platelet aggregation (sticky, clot-prone blood). EPA is found most abundantly in cold-water fatty fish.

Omega-6 (linoleic acid) comes from unprocessed vegetable oils (safflower, sunflower, corn and soy), nuts, seeds and wild game (especially game birds). In a healthy body, linoleic acid is converted into gamma-linolenic acid (GLA).

Like EPA, GLA is also converted in the body into beneficial prostaglandins. GLA-series prostaglandins widen blood vessels, keep blood platelets from sticking together, reduce inflammation and strengthen the immune system.

The best way to ensure a healthy balance of beneficial prostaglandins is to include both the Omega-3 rich oils and moderate amounts of Omega-6 oils in your daily diet. EPA in fish oil and GLA in borage oil are already in the form the body uses to produce the prostaglandin hormones.

Americans are both fat and Omega-fat deficient. We don't eat enough high quality Omega-3 and Omega-6 foods. Feedlot-raised cattle and caged chickens have up to five times less Omega-3 and Omega-6 fats than free-range cattle, chicken, sheep and wild game. The Omega-6 fats in commercially processed vegetable oils has been damaged by heat and chemicals in the refining process.

Damaged Vegetable Fats

Just as modern food processing has stripped carbohydrates of their fiber and nutritional value, fats have suffered a similar 20th century fate.

In 1910, Americans were preparing food with home-made vegetable oils cold-pressed in small batches. These minimally-processed oils were cloudy, dark in color and supplied Americans with many nutrients including vitamin E, vitamin B-6, magnesium, lecithin and essential fats – all missing in the modern supermarket cooking oils.

Advertised as "Cholesterol free" and "high in polyunsaturates," supermarket cooking oils – made from corn, sunflower, soy and safflower – are not safe for cooking.

When exposed to heat, light and air, fatty acids in these

oils are transformed from the natural "cis-configuration" to the not-found-in-nature "trans-configuration." Natural "cis-fats" melt at 55 degrees while altered "trans-fats" or TFAs melt at about 111 degrees – well above normal body temperature of 98.6.

In their altered state, these processed vegetable oils can't build healthy cell membranes. They also block conversion of natural fats into prostaglandins, upsetting the hormonal balance, increasing blood stickiness, and constricting arteries.

Crisco was introduced in the U.S. in 1911 by Proctor & Gamble. If you opened one of those cans today, chances are it would still be good. "Butterine," an early name for margarine, was introduced in the 1930s. It, too, had extended shelf life. In the 1950s, Minnesota and Wisconsin were the last two states to legalize colored margarine.

Margarine is a high TFA product made from refined vegetable oil that has been hydrogenated; that is, bombarded with hydrogen and high heat to make it "artificially saturated" – solid at room temperature. Hydrogenated (and partially hydrogenated) fats are found in thousands of supermarket products.

Peanut butters like Skippy® and Jif® contain partially hydrogenated fat, salt and a lot of sugar. They can sit in your cupboard for months. Most graham crackers, cookies, corn chips, salad dressings, dips, toppings, cakes and pancake mixes also contain plenty of sugar and hydrogenated oil. It's best to avoid these products altogether.

Today, margarine outsells butter. Butter is a pure, nutritionally-sound natural fat that has been used for thousands of years. The French, with the lowest heart disease rates in the Western world, use butter lavishly. According to Gittleman, the average American consumes 10 pounds of shortening and 20 pounds of margarine a year.

The Harvard School of Public Health's study of more than 85,000 nurses found a greater than 50 percent heart disease risk among those who ate high trans-fat foods such as margarine. Women who ate four or more teaspoons of margarine a day had a 66 percent greater risk of heart disease than women who ate less than one teaspoon a month.

Saturated animal fats, in moderation, are safer for cooking than the commercially processed vegetable oils.

Provided it does not burn (turn brown), butter is a safe cooking fat. Animal fats withstand high temperatures and remain chemically stable. Heating bacon fat, for example, does not generate trans-fatty acids.

There is no proof that saturated animal fats, as part of a healthy diet rich in nutrients and fiber, cause heart disease. In a low-fiber diet full of refined carbohydrates and damaged unsaturated vegetable oils, excess saturated animal fat can contribute to cellular degeneration, heart disease and heart failure.

Olive oil and avocado oil are heart-protective because they are stable fats for cooking. Produced throughout the world, olive oil has been used safely for 2,000 years. Classified as "monounsaturated," these oils are more stable at high temperatures and less prone to "oxidation" from heat, light and air than the Omega-6 polyunsaturated vegetable oils described previously.

Homogenization is another processing method that damages fat and extends shelf life. Normal milk fat occurs in large globules that are digested whole in the intestinal tract. Homogenization breaks up these fat globules into extremely small droplets, one-third their original size. Dispersed in milk, these small droplets bypass digestion and pass directly into the blood stream, carrying with them a destructive enzyme called xanthine oxidase (XO).

In the bloodstream, XO can irritate and injure artery walls. Chronic injury to artery walls may stimulate the over-production of cholesterol. Excess cholesterol can oxidize (break down) and adhere to artery walls.

Homogenized whole milk and 2% milk (which derives over 30 percent of its calories from fat) contain this damaged fat. Skim milk with 0 grams of fat does not. Finland has the highest per capita milk consumption and the highest death rate from heart disease, followed closely by the U.S.

Degenerative Disease Flourishes

The standard American diet delivers a destructive one-two punch. First, excess calories from highly processed foods replace calories from nutritious whole foods, causing subtle nutritional deficiencies that may go undetected for years.

According to medical researchers, deficiencies of magnesium, zinc, chromium, selenium and vitamins B_3, B_6, C and E have become widespread.

Second, without the nutritional environment provided by these missing nutrients, the hormonal balance needed for proper body functioning is not possible. In the absence of minerals, vitamins are not utilized by the body. In the absence of vital minerals like magnesium, zinc and chromium; dietary fats are less likely to convert in the body into the prostaglandin hormones. Without the essential fats and the nutrients required to produce the prostaglandin hormones, normal body function and circulation will be impaired.

Impaired circulation – over time – increases the heart's workload. The overburdened heart enlarges to compensate, further increasing its oxygen and nutrient requirements. Lacking sufficient nutrients, the heart's left ventricle progressively loses its ability to pump blood to the rest of the body. This is heart failure.

Heart failure is "multi-causal." Degeneration takes place over decades and is the result of a combination of dietary errors, including overeating; too much saturated and altered fat, lack of essential fatty acids; excess simple sugars and refined carbohydrates; and reliance on the denatured convenience foods that make up a high percentage of the calories in the standard American diet.

Denatured foods do cumulative damage. According to T.L Cleave, medical researcher and author of *The Saccharine Study*, diabetes, hypertension, varicose veins and heart disease appear about two decades after a culture begins consuming refined carbohydrates – sugar, corn syrup and white flour.

Heart disease was rare in 1910. By the '20s, "heart attack" was becoming medical jargon. In 1961, death from heart attack had reached a peak. Emergency Medical Treatment has since slowed the heart attack death rate, but the number of people with obesity, hypertension, diabetes, heart disease and heart failure is steadily increasing. Medical treatments for these conditions focus on managing the symptoms – not addressing the underlying causes.

Suppressing Symptoms

Instead of teaching us how to protect our bodies from cellular degeneration and hormonal imbalance, our medical system is geared toward managing disease symptoms with drugs. "My doctor says Mylanta," for example, may be masking serious digestive disorders that will ultimately result in chronic degenerative disease. Suppressing symptoms can be deadly.

Example: John Doe, age 50, visits his doctor for a routine physical. Tests show his blood cholesterol is 275 – an increase of 50 points from two years ago. He and the doctor are perplexed.

John switched to a low-fat, high carbohydrate diet two years ago. He has cut down on red meat, eats just 2-3 eggs a week, and has been dutifully eating margarine and "low-fat" foods for the past few years. John doesn't seem to notice that his "No-Fat" Snackwell® cookies are full of sugar and refined carbohydrates.

John is also eating a lot more pasta. He is gaining weight and feels tired all the time (too tired to exercise). For years, John ate too much saturated fat. He lunched daily at fast food restaurants. Now, he's cut back on fast foods, but he is eating a lot of refined carbohydrates, including plenty of sugar. His high insulin levels are raising dangerous blood fats (triglycerides) and elevating blood cholesterol levels.

John's doctor has decided to fight the cholesterol number itself. John's "anti-cholesterol" medication, Mevacor, works by interfering with liver function. Mevacor can reduce body stores of Coenzyme Q-10, an oxygen-sparing nutrient found most abundantly in heart muscle cells. A healthy body produces small amounts of Coenzyme Q-10.

Many people who suffer heart attacks are deficient in Coenzyme Q-10, magnesium, vitamin E and other essential nutrients. While anti-cholesterol drugs deplete enzymes, diuretic drugs like Lasix cause the body to lose potassium and magnesium.

Every day people like John are being treated with symptom-masking drugs that, all too often, hasten the very conditions they are prescribed to prevent. The drugs may work for a while, but eventually, because they do not harmonize with the delicate biochemistry of the human body, they exact their toll – sudden death.

John has a fatty acid deficiency. All he really needs is a daily tablespoon of fish oil and borage oil – and to stop eating damaged fat, sugar and refined carbohydrates.

The trans-fatty acids in the margarine and packaged food he is eating are preventing the natural fats in his diet from producing prostaglandins. His hormonal credit card is about to be revoked.

Upon arising on the morning of his 50th birthday, John fell dead of a heart attack. The coroner's report said he died of "natural causes." What could be further from the truth?

John died prematurely because he lived in a society that is out of touch – out of hormonal balance. The foods and drugs he was taking were artificial – not natural. They were designed to make money – not the strong, elastic arteries John needed to live his life to the fullest.

The Evils of Acidosis

In March 1995, Dick Quinn found himself on the verge of death, struggling with "late-stage" heart failure. Hospital blood work showed altered blood chemistry – high blood glucose and high levels of uric acid (a byproduct of protein metabolism); low levels of calcium, magnesium and sodium. His faulty diet – high in poor quality protein cooked in altered oils, excess sugar and simple carbohydrates – had brought him to the brink of "acidosis."

In Germany, cardiologists point to acidosis as the primary cause of heart disease. Heart attacks often occur in people with no arterial blockage. In the German view, chronic acidosis (accumulation of acid) and high blood viscosity (thickness) damage the heart's left ventricle, which pumps blood out to the body. The increased effort of circulating the thick, sticky blood makes the heart work even harder.

Acids are a normal byproduct of metabolizing carbohydrates, protein and fats. Because they are toxic to the kidney and liver, acid wastes must be neutralized by mineral compounds in the body before they are filtered out. Dietary excesses can overwhelm the body's ability to neutralize these strong acids. The cumulative effect of excess acids in the blood is the leaching of minerals, particularly calcium, from the bones.

Like body temperature, acid/alkaline balance in the blood is a constant the body must maintain. Blood must be slightly alkaline (pH 7.4) at all times. (pH 7 is neutral.) To maintain slightly alkaline blood, calcium may be summoned from the bone. Once mobilized to alkalize the blood, calcium cannot reenter the bone nor can it remain in the bloodstream. Instead, it is deposited in soft tissues like the cells of the muscles, arteries or heart.

Chronic acid conditions can cause calcium deficiencies in the bone and calcium saturation of soft tissue cells. This accumulation of calcium in heart muscle cells can cause heart attack, cardiac arrhythmia and sudden death. Calcium in the arteries can cause rigidity and constriction, increasing blood pressure and the possibility of fatal arterial spasms. In combination with coronary blockage and sticky clot-prone blood, arterial spasms can trigger a heart attack.

Although calcium is the most abundant mineral in the blood, magnesium is the most abundant mineral in soft tissue. Magnesium serves as the body's natural calcium-channel blocking agent. Magnesium prevents calcium accumulation in soft tissue cells by stimulating the production of a hormone, calcitonin, which increases calcium in the bones and keeps it from being absorbed into muscle cells.

Magnesium is the key mineral for heart health. It is an essential nutrient required for over 100 enzyme reactions in the body. In *Heart Healthy Magnesium*, James B. Pierce, Ph.D., refers to magnesium as the "biochemical gatekeeper."

Magnesium controls the concentrations of calcium, sodium and potassium in cells and surrounding fluids. Because magnesium controls the nervous system and neuro-muscular communications, low levels in the body magnify the risk of arterial spasms and cardiac arrhythmia, which can result in heart attack, and in time, heart failure.

The best way of maintaining sufficient bone calcium and a mineral balance is to eat magnesium-rich foods. Magnesium is found in whole grains, green vegetables, beans (especially soybeans), almonds, bananas, raisins, dates and seeds. Dehydrated seaweed contains exceptionally high concentrations of magnesium. Dairy, meat and eggs contain the least magnesium of common foods. Magnesium is depleted by alcohol, stress, sugar and the acids in coffee.

The remedy for acidosis is a whole foods diet containing

a wide variety of high quality fruits and alkaline-forming vegetables. High quality protein, complex carbohydrates and natural fats would be balanced in each meal. This diet would not include any refined carbohydrates, damaged fats or processed foods. For people suffering with acidosis-related heart failure, specific macrobiotic foods may offer the greatest therapeutic benefit.

The Macrobiotic Approach

With humility and self-effacing humor, Dick Quinn entered the world of macrobiotics. In the same spirit he began other new ventures, he immediately went out and bought *Diet For A Strong Heart* by Michio Kushi, *Acid & Alkaline* by Herman Aihara and two new macrobiotic cookbooks. It wasn't long before he was enjoying seaweed and soybean paste, brown rice and green tea, gomashio and umeboshi plum concentrate.

There is no one macrobiotic diet; instead, it is a unique way of cooking and meal-planning based on principles that emphasize preventing disease through diet. As Dick learned, macrobiotic foods can be used by those already ill to promote healing or at least improve the quality of life. People close to Dick saw a dramatic improvement as he incorporated whole foods into his diet.

Cooked whole grains, like short grain brown rice, are a macrobiotic staple. Brown rice is gluten-free (a common allergen found in wheat), easy to digest if chewed well, and a concentrated source of B-vitamins. Like magnesium, B-vitamins perform numerous tasks in the body and are easily depleted by alcohol, stress and refined carbohydrates.

Brown rice is also mineral-rich (magnesium, selenium, iron and zinc) and contains three times more fiber than white rice. Brown rice combines better with animal protein (fish, fowl and beef) than gluten-rich starches like whole wheat.

Used as a soup base and seasoning for 2,500 years, miso is a protein-rich fermented soybean paste that contains an amino acid pattern and hearty flavor similar to meat. Unpasteurized, miso is an enzyme-rich food that contains a lactobacillus (like the bacteria in yogurt) that aids in digestion. Miso creates an alkaline condition in the body and provides a trace of vitamin B_{12}.

Miso is very concentrated. A little goes a long way. People with heart failure should use the lighter, less fermented variety. In moderate amounts – one bowl daily – miso soup can help balance acid conditions created by eating too much sugar, meat and grain-based carbohydrates.

Miso soup is prepared with a variety of ingredients, including burdock root, carrot, daikon radish, eggplant, leek, white and green onions, tofu, turnip and seaweed.

A long, thin dried seaweed, wakame is a standard ingredient in basic miso soup (1/2 cup chopped into small pieces). Sea vegetables are alkaline-forming foods and wakame is the most alkaline-forming of all. High in calcium, niacin and thiamine, wakame is the most concentrated source of magnesium on earth – second only to Hijiki, another seaweed.

Seaweeds, sardines, almonds, parsley, sunflower seeds, garbanzo beans, black beans, pistachios, pinto beans and spirulina all contain more calcium than milk. These foods also contain high concentrations of magnesium, forming a calcium/magnesium balance that is in harmony with the body's own mineral requirements. In contrast, milk is relatively high in calcium but low in magnesium. Also, food processing has rendered the nutrients in milk less available and even dangerous to your health.

People wanting to extend their life – especially those with heart failure – should strongly consider incorporating some of these ancient macrobiotic principles into their cooking and meal planning.

For more information or a referral to a macrobiotic counselor, write to Kushi Institute, PO Box 7, Becket, MA 01223 or call (413) 623-5741.

Food Choices

Dick had more than his share of red meat – which contributed to his heart failure. However, a healing diet isn't necessarily meatless. Constitutionally weak people can benefit from high quality red meat and some people need more meat than others.

Although some people thrive on a low-fat, high carbohydrate diet, others on the same diet will slow down physically and mentally. Not everyone can be a vegetarian, although most Americans would benefit from eating more vegetarian foods. Whether or not meat consumption is healthful depends on your genes, other foods and nutrients in your diet, and the quality of the meat you select.

Meat is best in small portions (2-4 oz.), oven-roasted and served with plenty of vegetables. Eggs, chicken, fish, lamb and beef can be wholesome sources of protein, zinc and all other minerals. Lean organic meats or wild game contain few if any toxins, hormones and antibiotics. Prepared, aged or fried meat such as sausage, lunch meat and hamburger contain oxidized cholesterol, nitrates and other harmful ingredients.

According to Dr. Cass Igram in *Eat Right To Live Long*, the heart muscle loves fat, efficiently metabolizing it into energy. Lamb fat is loaded with carnitine (L-Carnitine), an amino acid that promotes fat burning. Carnitine enhances the delivery of fatty acids into heart muscle cells. Lamb meat and fat are the richest known sources of carnitine unless they are overcooked. Avocado is the richest plant source followed by cauliflower and cabbage.

Animal protein foods, in moderation, are also good sources of amino acids like taurine. Just as carnitine carries fat into the cell membrane, taurine carries minerals to the cells and locks them up. Taurine is synthesized by the liver from the amino acid cysteine. Cysteine is found in a wide variety of animal protein foods.

Dr. Atkins recommends giving supplemental taurine to heart failure patients as a diuretic. Supplementing individual amino acids is best done under the guidance of a nutritionally-oriented physician.

Eggs contain all eight essential amino acids. That's why eggs are considered a perfect food. However, eggs are a common allergen and can create a thick mucus condition in some people.

If you can eat eggs, they are good for you – again, in moderation and properly prepared. If they're overcooked or not fresh, they're not good for you. Free range chicken eggs contain 10 times more lecithin than commercially raised eggs, which contain little or no vitamin B_{12} and are lacking in virtually every other nutrient. Poached or soft-boiled eggs retain the lecithin in the yolk. Dried eggs and milk in packaged food products contain very high levels of oxidized (damaged) cholesterol.

Grains have unique and widely different natures. Wheat, rye, oats and barley contain gluten, the sticky protein portion of the grain. Gluten-containing refined grains and flour products are the predominant American carbohydrate food.

An excessively gluten-based diet of refined carbohydrates is not only nutrient-poor, but also promotes mineral and vitamin deficiencies, intestinal inflammation and allergic reactions. In adults, skin conditions like eczema have been linked to gluten intolerance. According to Gittleman, the B-vitamins, especially folic acid and vitamin B_{12}, are not well absorbed in a gluten-irritated intestinal lining.

Non-gluten grains include: millet, corn, rice, quinoa, amaranth and buckwheat. Millet helps balance over-acid conditions; fresh corn on the cob is vitamin and enzyme-rich; brown rice is especially high in niacin; amaranth is excellent for pregnant and nursing women and those who do heavy physical work; rutin, in buckwheat strengthens arterial walls.

Discovering the right grains for you can enhance your cardiovascular health. However, most Americans cannot identify whole-wheat berries, brown rice, barley, rye or buckwheat, nor do we know how to prepare or chew them. We grew up wolfing down refined grains in the form of flour products, instant oatmeal, white rice and highly processed breakfast cereals.

To benefit from the nutritional bounty of whole cereal grains – without suffering from gas, bloating and intestinal distress – they must be introduced gradually into the diet and chewed thoroughly for complete digestion. Macrobiotic cookbooks are a good resource for learning how to prepare nutritious, good-tasting grains.

While meat-based protein and grain-based carbohydrates must be balanced in the diet, vegetables are excellent companions to all foods (except fruit which should be eaten alone). You can't go wrong eating unprocessed and unimproved fresh vegetables such as artichoke, asparagus, beets, broccoli, brussels sprouts, cabbage, carrots, cauliflower, celery, corn, eggplant, endive, garlic, green beans, lettuce, onions, parsnips, peppers, tomatoes, turnips, sprouts and zucchini.

Eating a wide variety of vegetables every day will help provide vitamins and minerals as well as soluble fiber. Organic, in season, and locally grown are best. Serving vegetables with grains or protein foods provides more complete nourishment. Properly prepared vegetables provide enzymes and fiber that help detoxify the body.

Vegetables are a vital part of the daily diet. Like grains, vegetables have widely different natures. *Healing With Whole Foods*, by Paul Pitchford, and various vegetarian cookbooks highlight these differences.

Cabbage, for example, comes in green and purple varieties. Like broccoli, cabbage has potent antioxidant activity. Eaten raw or steamed, cabbage improves digestion, benefiting the stomach and intestines. Cabbage in the form of raw sauerkraut is especially beneficial for the digestive tract, rejuvenating intestinal flora. Drinking freshly made cabbage juice two or three times a day between meals can help heal stomach or duodenal ulcers.

Cabbage has a high sulfur content. Sulfur purifies the blood and destroys parasites. Eating cabbage and garlic together can help rid the digestive system of worms. Cabbage contains high amounts of vitamin C (more than oranges) concentrated in the core of the plant, which is not destroyed in storage, cooking or in making sauerkraut.

Vegetables are excellent nutritional partners for whole grains and protein. But, like a lot else in diet and nutrition, the importance of "food combinations" will vary from person to person.

However, there are some basic rules that seem to apply to everyone. Fruit should be eaten alone as refreshing snacks or energizing meals. Drink milk alone. Proteins, fats and starches combine best with green and non-starchy vegetables. A lamb chop is best with vegetables, sparing the potato or pasta. In a combination meal, eat the highest protein food first. Protein requires a lot of stomach acid; starches and vegetables do not.

Too much food at a meal and too many different types of food challenge the digestive system. People with healthy digestion may ignore some of the food combining rules. People with heart failure will greatly benefit from eating simple meals that do not combine protein and starch, such as meat and potatoes.

PART THREE: THREE STEPS TO HEART HEALTH

A Flicker of Warning

At age 42, on a chilly May evening in Somerset, Wisconsin, Dick Quinn felt angina pains while chasing around in the dark after the family steer. He couldn't believe it was actually happening to him.

Today, millions of Americans are heading Dick's way, discovering, as he did, that in the very prime of life, life may be taken away. Like the film flickering in the best part of a thrilling movie, the spell of life is easily broken. A break in the film; a dangerous blood clot in a clogged artery and everything changes.

Dick Quinn shared his wake-up call with the rest of us. He took action. He put Cayenne in his mouth and his clogged arteries cleared, his angina disappeared and his fears of another heart attack abated. "This," Dick would say, "really got my attention."

By 1988, Dick was in the herbal supplement business. He was the first person to put fiery African Cayenne into a capsule. He manufactured a variety of herbal formulas with Cayenne as captain of the team.

In April 1992, when sales reached $1 million a year, Dick gave away his herb business to publish *Left For Dead*. His message was: Take Cayenne and avoid the surgeon's knife and the doctor's drugs.

In celebration of his victory over that hated enemy – death – Dick Quinn went out and told the world all about it. But needs change over time. In 1978, Cayenne was all he needed to feel good but as the years went by his needs changed. He simply did not know that what he was eating was slowly killing him.

To prevent heart failure, eliminating bad foods from the diet is the first order of business. Healing starts by eliminating the causes of disease.

Excess refined flour, white sugar, altered fats, poor quality meat and the many additives and chemicals in our food supply contribute significantly to heart disease. Until these negative foods are eliminated from our diet, optimum body functioning and long-term good health are not possible.

Don't put toxins in the body, and the body won't have to work overtime getting rid of them – driving up blood pressure, shifting blood sugars and leaching minerals from the bone to balance blood acids.

For example, in Chinese medicine, the liver is said to control blood pressure. The greater the detoxification demand on the liver, the greater its fresh blood requirement. A liver with a demanding schedule will increase blood pressure in order to assure itself sufficient blood for detoxification. When the liver's workload lightens, so will its demand for blood.

The second priority is replacing harmful altered foods with high quality natural foods. Whole grains replace refined flour. Extra virgin olive oil should replace refined vegetable oils. Fresh fish should replace fish sticks. Organic vegetables should replace pesticide-laden vegetables. A baked potato should replace French fries. Eating leisurely, wholesome meals with family or friends should replace the fast food drive-thru.

The third priority is to determine your own nutrient needs. Once you know where you stand and what you need, you can supplement any deficiencies with strengthening and toning remedies. Herbs are both nutrient-dense natural foods and medicinal remedies. Used wisely, herbs can help stimulate, cleanse, strengthen and tone (build) the cells, tissues and organs of the body. Herbal supplements are easily recognized and absorbed by the body.

Medicinal herbs work best when we have eliminated the harmful foods (and negative habits) from our diet. Otherwise, we are burning down our house and spraying water on it at the same time. This will work for a while as it did for Dick Quinn. But, in time, we weaken the body's self-regulating mechanisms, the fire reaches the rafters and our house comes tumbling down.

Though natural foods and herbs should be our first line of defense against heart failure, nutritional supplements can play an important role in closing nutritional gaps. Building resistance to disease depends on the interaction of a wide range of nutrients. The way antioxidants work illustrates nutritional teamwork.

Recently, a well-publicized study concluded that beta carotene was ineffective against cancer. In the study, a large group of physicians took synthetic beta carotene every other day for two years without any proof that it reduced their incidence of cancer. Of course not.

Antioxidants work as a team. Sending beta carotene out by itself against cancer is like sending a baseball team out on the field with only a pitcher. With eight missing players, the home team is going to lose.

Beta carotene, vitamin C, vitamin E and the minerals zinc, copper, manganese and selenium are antioxidants. Antioxidants prevent oxygen free radicals from damaging cholesterol in the blood. Cholesterol, a beneficial substance, can no longer soothe and heal artery walls when it has been altered. Instead, oxidized cholesterol, like damaged cooking fats, injures artery walls.

Supplemental sources of beta carotene, vitamin C, vitamin E, zinc, copper, manganese and selenium work best when combined. Although the best sources of antioxidants are organic foods, there is evidence that sufficient levels of vitamin C and vitamin E can only be achieved in supplemental form. In larger dosages, nutritional supplements become natural therapeutic agents.

Supplemental vitamin E helps prevent the oxidation of cholesterol and dangerous blood clots from forming. The Harvard Medical School study cited earlier found that nurses who supplemented with at least 100 IUs of vitamin E daily for more than two years had a 46 percent lower risk of heart disease. A minimum of 400 IUs daily of natural vitamin E (d-alpha tocopherol) is recommended for people with existing cardiovascular disease. Synthetic vitamin E, made from petroleum, is the least active.

Like vitamin E, vitamin C prevents free radical oxidation of cholesterol. Studies also reveal that vitamin C produces the collagen that keeps artery walls elastic. A deficiency of vitamin C can result in injury to arterial walls.

Vitamin C also enhances the action of vitamin E and iron absorption. A minimum of 500 milligrams of vitamin C (in the mineral ascorbate form with bioflavonoids) twice a day is recommended for people with existing cardiovascular disease.

B-vitamins, like the mineral magnesium, are "energy" nutrients – they are the catalysts that turn food into energy. Whole grains contain B-vitamins (brown rice is the most concentrated source). Like vitamin C, B-vitamins are water soluble (not stored in the body) and must be replenished daily. Because B-vitamins function together, a supplement should include the entire B-complex. Alcohol, stress and sugar can easily deplete both B-vitamins and magnesium.

Recent studies have shown that vitamins B_6, B_{12}, and folic acid can dramatically lower homocysteine levels in the blood. Homocysteine is a potent free radical generator that damages cholesterol and directly injures artery walls. Optimal levels of these B-vitamins convert homocysteine into a harmless chemical that is then removed from the body. Dr. Robert Atkins recommends a combination of folic acid (5-10 mg), vitamin B_{12} (500-600 mcg), and vitamin B_6 (200-300 mg) for patients with existing heart disease.

Supplemental sources of magnesium and calcium should be taken in a one-to-one ratio (as they are found naturally in foods such as dried sea vegetables, sardines, nuts and seeds). People with existing heart disease may need to supplement with more magnesium than calcium. Sufficient tissue levels of magnesium can prevent unwanted calcium from accumulating in artery walls, reducing the chance of "hardening" of the arteries and high blood pressure.

Like antioxidants, minerals function interactively in the body. Too much of one mineral, such as calcium, can lead to a general mineral imbalance. Because magnesium regulates the concentrations of calcium and other major minerals, a mineral balance cannot be achieved if magnesium levels are low.

Overcoming his own life-threatening magnesium deficiency, James B. Pierce, Ph.D., author of *Heart Healthy Magnesium*, recommends that if you supplement with just one mineral, make it magnesium. Recent studies reveal that individuals who die suddenly of heart attack have far lower levels of magnesium (and potassium) than normal. Magnesium helps to dilate arteries and ease the heart's pumping of blood, effectively preventing irregular heartbeats (arrhythmias).

Magnesium oxide is the least expensive and most poorly absorbed form. It is estimated that healthy people absorb no more than 40 percent of magnesium oxide. People with impaired digestion or low levels of stomach acid may absorb very little. Magnesium aspartate is more effective than the oxide. Aspartic acid "delivers" magnesium into the cell membrane where it is absorbed, and then chelates (or carries out) unwanted excess calcium that has been deposited into cells and tissues.

All minerals are important for heart health – even trace minerals. Selenium, for example, is an important antioxidant that is deficient in many of our soils.

The best sources of trace minerals are organic fruits and vegetables, whole grains, fish, high quality meats and mineral-rich water. Liquid "ionic" trace mineral supplements are ideal since they are in a form that doesn't require stomach acid for absorption. If you supplement trace minerals, it's best to choose a product that contains all of them.

A deficiency of Coenzyme Q10 is also common in people with heart disease. CoQ10, a close relative of the B-vitamins, helps to strengthen the heart muscle by enhancing the ability of heart cells to use oxygen more efficiently. CoQ10 is found in every cell of the body and is the key catalyst in producing cellular energy. The greatest concentration of CoQ10 is found in heart muscle cells.

Since the heart is the most metabolically active organ in the body, it is the most sensitive to CoQ10 deficiency. As we age or fall victim to nutritional deficiencies, our body's production of CoQ10 declines. CoQ10 supplements are recommended by nutritional doctors in ranges from 30 milligrams daily as a maintenance dose, up to 200-300 milligrams for people with congestive heart failure. CoQ10 is safe and non-toxic in these doses.

L-Carnitine, the supplemental form of the amino acid carnitine, is often recommended by nutritional doctors to be used in conjunction with Coenzyme Q-10 to prevent heart disease or to treat heart failure. L-Carnitine transports fats into the cell membrane where they are metabolized as fuel for energy production. By increasing heart cell energy production, the heart pumps blood more efficiently. L-Carnitine is recommended in ranges of 600-1,000 milligrams.

Since most Americans are deficient in essential fat, daily supplements will help ensure stable cell membranes and balanced hormone production. Daily doses of essential fats will also increase levels of beneficial HDL cholesterol while lowering both LDL cholesterol (so-called "bad" cholesterol) and triglycerides (other fats traveling in the blood).

Gamma linolenic acid (GLA) in Borage Oil and EPA in fish oil should be taken in a one-to-one ratio according to Dr. Atkins, in the range of 800-1,600 milligrams daily. Other excellent sources of fatty acids include milled flax seed (2 tablespoons a day) and lecithin granules (2 table-spoons a day).

Dosages of nutritional supplements vary according to age, sex, weight, diet, use of prescription drugs and state of health. Too little or too much can stress the body.

Natural foods, medicinal herbs and high quality supple-ments can help prevent heart failure. If you have heart fail-ure, a combination of timely self-study, nutritional counsel-ing and the services of a nutritionally-oriented physician can help you extend and improve the quality of your life.

Circulation is life itself. Good circulation can help you live your life to the fullest and it's never too late to improve it. As Dick Quinn wrote in *Left For Dead*, "Take charge of your health. Make your own decisions. You're worth saving."

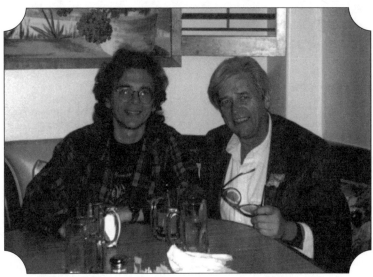

AL WATSON AND DICK QUINN RELAX AT THE TROPICANA BAR AND GRILL IN SAN CLEMENTE, CALIF. IN JANUARY 1995 – ONE MONTH AFTER DICK WAS DIAGNOSED WITH END-STAGE CONGESTIVE HEART FAILURE.

BIBLIOGRAPHY

**Books used for Herbal section
"Medicines of the Meadow:"**

The Doctors' Vitamin and Mineral Encyclopedia, Sheldon Saul Hendler, MD, Ph.D., 1990, Fireside Press, New York, NY.

School of Natural Healing, Dr. John R. Christopher, 1976, Christopher Publications, Inc., Springville, Utah

The Way of Herbs, Michael Tierra, C.A., ND, 1983, Washington Square Press, New York, NY.

The Scientific Validation of Herbal Medicine, Daniel B. Mowrey, Ph.D., 1986, Cormorant Books.

Next Generation Herbal Medicine, Revised Edition, Daniel B. Mowrey, Ph.D., 1988, Cormorant Books, 1990, Keats Publishing, Inc., New Canaan, CT.

Proven Herbal Blends: A Rational Approach to Prevention and Remedy, Daniel B. Mowrey, Ph.D., 1986, Keats Publishing, Inc., New Canaan, CT.

Herbal Tonic Therapies, Daniel B. Mowrey, Ph.D., 1993, Keats Publishing, Inc., New Canaan, CT.

An Elders' Herbal: Natural Techniques for Promoting Health and Vitality, David Hoffmann, 1993, Healing Arts Press, Rochester, VT.

The Herbal Handbook: A User's Guide to Medical Herbalism; David Hoffmann, 1987, Healing Arts Press, Rochester, VT.

The Elements of Herbalism, David Hoffmann, 1991, Element, Inc., Rockport, MA.

Indian Herbalogy of North America, Alma R. Hutchens, 1973, Shambhala Publications, Inc., Boston, MA.

How to be Your Own Herbal Pharmacist, Linda Rector-Page ND, Ph.D., 1991.

Natural Healing With Herbs, Humbart Santillo, Hohm Press, Prescott, AZ.

Chinese Herbs, John D. Keys, 1976, Charles E. Tuttle Company, Inc., Bunkyo-ku, Tokyo.

Healing with Herbs, Henrietta A. Diers Rau, 1968, Arco Publishing, Inc., New York, NY.

Left For Dead, Dick Quinn, 1992, R.F. Quinn Publishing Co., Minneapolis, MN.

The Complete Medicinal Herbal, Penelope Ody, 1993, Dorling Kindersley, Inc., New York, NY.

The Vitamin Herb Guide, 1987, Global Health, Ltd., Alberta, Canada.

Herbs & Things, Jeanne Rose, 1972, Grosset & Dunlap, Workman Publishing Co., New York, NY.

The Complete Herbalist, Dr. O. Phelps Brown, 1993, Newcastle Publishing Company, Inc., Van Nuys, CA.

Modern Herbal, Vols I and II, Mrs. M. Grieve, 1971, Dover Publishing, New York, NY.

The Illustrated Encyclopedia of Herbs, Jiri Stodola and Jan Volak, 1992, Chancellor Press, London.

The Food Pharmacy, Jean Carper,

1988, Bantam Books, New York, NY.

Nature's Medicines, Richard Lucas, Parker Publications, West Nyack, NY.

Rondale's Illustrated Encyclopedia of Herbs, Rodale Press, Emmaus, PA.

The A to Z Guide to Herbal Healing Remedies, Jason Elias, MA L.Ac. and Shelagh Ryan Masline, 1995, Dell Publishing, New York, NY.

Earl Mindell's Herb Bible, Earl Mindell, R.Ph., Ph.D. and Carol Colman, 1992, Simon & Schuster/Fireside, New York, NY.

The Herbs of Life: Health and Healing Using Western and Chinese Techniques, Leslie Tierra, L.Ac., Herbalist, 1992, Crossing Press, Freedom, CA.

Sources for "Anatomy of a Killer" and "Medical Approaches to Heart Failure:"

The American Heart Association Heart Book, 1980, Dutton Publishers, New York, NY.

Conquering Heart Disease: New Ways to Live Well Without Drugs or Surgery, Harvey B. Simon, MD, 1994, Little, Brown & Co., New York, NY.

Mayo Clinic Heart Book: The Ultimate Guide to Heart Health, 1993, Mayo Foundation for Medical Education and Research, William Morrow & Co., New York, NY.

Yale University School of Medicine Heart Book, Medical Editors: Barry L. Zaret MD, Lawrence Cohen MD, Marvin Moser MD, 1992, Hearst Books, New York, NY.

Success With Heart Failure: Help and Hope For Those With Congestive

Heart Failure, Marc A. Silver MD, 1994, Insight Books, Plenum Publishing, New York, NY.

Worst Pills Best Pills II, Sidney M. Wolfe, MD, Rose-Ellen Hope, R.Ph., 1993, Public Citizen Health Research Group, Washington D.C.

The Handbook of Heart Drugs: A Consumer's Guide to Safe and Effective Use, Martin Goldman, MD, 1992, Henry Holt and Co., New York, NY.

Deadly Medicine: Why tens of thousands of heart patients died in America's worst drug disaster, Thomas J. Moore, 1995, Simon and Schuster, New York, NY.

Books used for the diet section "Fueling the Fight Against Heart Failure:"

Acid & Alkaline Revised, Herman Aihara, 1986, George Ohsawa Macrobiotic Foundation, Oroville, CA.

Beyond Pritikin, Ann Louise Gittleman, MS, 1988, Bantam Books, New York, NY.

Diet For A Strong Heart, Michio Kushi, 1985, St. Martin's Press, New York, NY.

Dr. Atkins' New Diet Revolution, Robert Atkins, MD, 1992, M. Evans & Co., New York, NY.

Enter The Zone, Barry Sears, Ph.D., 1995, HarperCollins, New York, NY.

Heart Healthy Magnesium, James B. Pierce, Ph.D., 1994, Avery, Garden City Park, NY.

Optimal Wellness, Ralph Golan, MD, 1995, Ballantine Books, New York, NY.

The Facts About Fats, John Finnegan, 1993, Celestial Books, Berkley, CA.

GLOSSARY / INDEX

Acidosis: Abnormal state of reduced alkalinity of blood and tissues. Acidosis thickens the blood and builds up acids or toxins in the heart muscle cells. *63, 65, 162, 199-201*

Adaptogen: A term coined for Ginseng. An adaptogen helps the body cope with emotional and physical stress by normalizing body functions. *155-157*

Aneurysm: Balloon-like swelling of arterial wall. *102-103, 162, 164, 182*

Angiogram: A procedure in which a narrow tube called a catheter is threaded through the arteries to the heart. *77*

Angioplasty: An operation in which a balloon-tipped catheter is inflated to compact plaque against the artery walls. *62, 101*

Antispasmodic: Antispasmodic herbs relieve muscle spasms and ease muscle tension. Some antispasmodic herbs also alleviate nervous tension. *124, 140, 142, 144, 145*

Arrhythmia: Disrupted heart rhythm. The heart may beat too fast, too slow or skip beats. *12, 57-58, 66-67, 75, 80-84, 88-90, 95, 99-100, 107-108, 112, 120, 124, 137-139, 155, 158, 200, 209*

Aorta: The main trunk of the arterial system carrying blood from the heart to the rest of the body. *43, 100, 102, 184*

Arteries: Muscular tubes that carry oxygenated blood throughout the body. *17-18, 43, 46, 48, 50, 60, 62-65, 78, 82, 85, 90-91, 99-102, 106, 110, 112-114, 120-121, 124-125, 128, 140, 144, 148, 153, 163, 168, 183, 186, 188, 190, 193, 195, 199-200, 206, 208*

Arterioles: Small branches off the arteries that funnel the blood down into the capillaries. *46, 49, 91*

Asymptomatic Stage: The stage of CHF where there are no visible symptoms and the body is attempting to compensate for a weak heart. *44, 46, 50, 57*

Atherosclerosis: The formation of plaque in the arteries. *62-63, 66, 102*

Atrioventricular Node (*AV Node*): Part of the heart's conduction system. *56*

Atrium: The two smaller chambers of the heart, located on the upper part of the heart. *42-43, 48, 56, 83*

Bitter: The taste of bitter herbs triggers the production of digestive hormones that stimulate the flow of digestive juices and bile; increase appetite and help detoxify the liver. *117-118, 124, 142, 149-150, 170*

Blood Pressure: The resistance of blood to flowing through the body. *42, 46, 49-52, 58-62, 64, 67, 71, 73-74, 82-83, 86-91, 94-97, 102-103, 106, 108, 110, 112, 114-115, 119-121, 123-138, 140-149, 153-158, 163-164, 168, 170, 172, 184, 186-187, 190, 200, 207, 209*

Bradycardia:When the heart skips a beat or beats less frequently than it should. *58-59, 128*

Capillaries: Microscopically thin passages in which the blood deposits oxygen and nutrients within the body's tissues and removes waste products. *46, 48, 50-51, 60, 64-65, 114, 120, 124-125, 132, 139, 162-164*

Cardiomyoplasty: An experimental procedure in which a muscle is taken from another part of a person's body – usually their back – and used as a supplemental heart muscle. *98*

Cardioversion: To correct an arrhythmia by stopping, then restarting the beat in sync to the natural rhythm with a carefully timed shock of the heart muscle. *19-20, 98-100*

Cardiac Output *(CO)*: The total amount of blood pumped by the heart in one minute. *70, 86, 99*

Cholesterol: A fatty substance found in all tissue of the body. It is contained in animal fat, produced by the body and carried in the bloodstream as lipoprotein. Oxidized cholesterol has been damaged by heat, light, oxygen and free radicals. *110,*

120, 125-126, 128-129, 130-131, 140, 148, 152-153, 155, 157, 169, 184-187, 189, 192, 194, 196, 198, 203-204, 208, 211

Congestive Heart Failure *(CHF)*: A condition in which the heart cannot pump enough blood to meet the body's needs.

Decoction: A medicinal tea made by boiling herbs in water. Used for harder plants, woody stems, seeds and course bark. *116-118*

Demulcent: Herbs that soothe the inflamed tissues of the bladder, kidney and liver. *167*

Dilated Cardiomyopathy: An enlargement of the heart chambers in response to inadequate blood flow in the body caused by heart failure. *47*

Diuretics: A class of high blood pressure drugs that rid the body of excess water. *80, 85, 87-89, 92, 107, 111-112, 114, 120, 124, 130-131, 134, 140, 142, 149-150, 152, 158-160, 162-163, 165-172, 174*

Dyspnea: Shortness of breath. *49*

Echocardiogram: test that uses sound waves to construct an image of the heart. *70-71, 76*

Edema: The buildup of excess fluid primarily in the legs and lower abdomen. *44, 51, 54, 57*

Eicosapentaenoic acid *(EPA)*: The Omega-3 essential fatty acid found primarily in cold-water fish. *194, 211*

Electrocardiogram *(ECG)*: A test which measures the electrical activity of the heart. *71, 74*

Essential fatty acids: A fatty acid the body cannot manufacture and must obtain from foods. Includes Omega-3 (from cold water fatty fish and flax seed), Omega-6 (from vegetable and botanical sources), and Gamma-linolenic-acid (GLA). *193, 197*

Extracts: Herbal extracts use solvents to extract the major components from the herb. These extracts are up to 10 times more concentrated than ordinary tinctures. *118, 127, 134, 139*

Fibrin: A chemical called fibrin causes the blood to clot. Too much fibrin can cause deadly clots to form. The process of ridding the body of excess fibrin is called fibrinosis. Herbs such as Cayenne stimulate fibrinosis. *126, 130, 150*

Free radical: A highly reactive chemical compound created by radiation, environmental toxins, heat and chemical processing of foods, and normal body metabolic functions. *187, 208-209*

Gamma-linolenic acid *(GLA)*: A fatty acid often considered essential. Found in borage, black current and evening primrose oil. Produces prostaglandin hormones. *194, 211*

Glucagon: A protein-induced hormone that balances insulin by increasing blood sugar levels and mobilizing fats from storage

tissue. *190-191*

Glucose: A simple sugar. The body's primary energy fuel (blood sugar). *189-192, 199*

Gluten: The sticky, protein portion of cereal grains. *201, 204*

Glycemic index: The entry rate of a carbohydrate into the bloodstream. The lower the glycemic index, the slower the rate of absorption. *189-190, 192-193*

Heart Attack: The death of a portion of heart muscle caused by either the buildup of acidity in the cells or a blockage of the coronary arteries that feed the affected area.

Hematocrit Level: The viscosity or thickness of the blood.

Hepatomegaly: The pooling of fluid in the liver which starves the organ causing it to sicken. *53*

Homocysteine: A dangerous substance that can injure the arteries and increase the risk of heart attack. *209*

Homogenization: A milk-processing method whereby fat globules are broken down into smaller particles one-third their original size. *196*

Hormone: A chemical compound that regulates many vital body functions. *189-190, 193-194, 196-197, 200, 203, 210*

Hydrogenated fat: An unsaturated fat, usually a vegetable oil, that has been processed with high heat and hydrogen to make it hard. Margarine and shortening are made from hydrogenated fats. *195*

Hypertrophic Cardiomyopathy: One of the heart's compensation methods, this condition is characterized by a thickening of the heart muscle. *46*

Hypoglycemia: Low blood sugar. *191-192*

Hypotensive: Herbs that lower high blood pressure. *135, 142, 144, 152, 172*

Infusion: A strong medicinal tea made by steeping herbs in hot water. Infusions are used for powdered herbs or delicate plant parts such as leaves, flowers and soft stems and those with delicate volatile oils. *115-119*

Insulin: A hormone produced by the pancreas that metabolizes blood sugar, converting it to energy or storing it as fat. *166, 186, 189-192, 198*

Lipid: A fat, oil or fat-like substance such as cholesterol.

Lipoprotein: Molecule combining protein and fat, allowing substances that are insoluble in the blood to circulate through the body. *128, 130, 186*

Macrobiotic: A way of cooking that helps prevent heart disease by restoring blood alkalinity. Developed by Japanese philosopher George Ohsawa. *201-202, 204*

Miso: Fermented soybean paste eaten in Japan and China for 2,500 years. Noted in macrobiotic cooking as alkaline-producing in the body. *201-202*

Monounsaturated fat: A non-essential fatty acid valued as a source of stable cooking fats, such as olive, sesame and almond oils. *196*

Myocardial Infarction: See Heart Attack.

Nocturia: When pooled blood starts to circulate in a more normal fashion through the kidneys. This occurs when a person with circulatory problems lies in a horizontal position - usually after they go to sleep at night. *52*

Omega-3 fatty acid: Linolenic acid contained in seed oils like flax and cold-water fish. *193-194, 196*

Omega-6 fatty acid: Linoleic acid found in vegetable and seed oils like sunflower, safflower and corn. *192, 194, 196*

pH: A scale from 0 to 14 used in measuring the acidity or alkalinity of solutions. Pure water, at pH 7.0, is considered neutral. Normal blood pH is 7.4. Acidity increases as the numbers decrease.

Plasma: A clear fluid, mostly made up of water, that carries the blood cells through the body. *42, 50-51, 64*

Polyunsaturated fat: Fats derived from vegetable and marine oils. *196*

Prostaglandin: Short-lived hormones derived from essential fatty acids that regulate body functions. *193-195, 197, 199*

Saturated fat: A type of fat solid at room temperature. Found mainly in meat, butter, coconut oil and palm kernel oil. *188, 192, 196-198*

Sinus Node: Part of the heart's conduction system where the impulses that cause the heart to contract originate. *56*

Stroke Volume: The amount of blood pumped out of the heart with each stroke or beat. *70*

Synergistic herbs: Herbs that have greater effect when combined than they do separately. An example would be Cayenne and Garlic. *110, 113*

Tinctures: Herbal alcohol and water concentrates. Stronger than infusions and decoctions, tinctures are taken by the drop or teaspoon. *111, 115-119*

Trans fatty acid *(TFA):* Natural cis-fats that have been chemically transformed by high heat or chemicals during processing. TFAs do not produce prostaglandin hormones and are biochemically useless. *195-196, 199*

Triglycerides: Fats circulating in the blood. *189, 198, 211*

Unsaturated fatty acid: Fats that are liquid at room temperature. Found in nuts, fish and vegetable oils. Unsaturated fats are mono- or poly-unsaturated, depending on their molecular makeup. Essential fatty acids are polyunsaturated. *193*

Vascular: Pertaining to the blood vessels or the circulatory system as a whole. *184, 188*

Vasodilator: Drugs or herbs that reduce high blood pressure by preventing constriction of the blood vessels. *88, 90, 95, 113, 120, 129-130, 134, 140, 146, 152, 154*

Veins: Tubes that carry blood from the body back to the heart to be oxygenated.

Ventricle: The two larger chambers of the heart which do the majority of the work, pushing the blood out into the body or to the lungs. *42-43, 46, 48, 50-51, 56, 59*

Wakame: A sea vegetable or seaweed noted in Japan for its high concentration of magnesium, calcium and other minerals. *202*

MEASUREMENTS

1 ounce = 28.3 grams

1 quart = 2 pints

1 pint = 2 cups

1 cup = 8 ounces

1 fluid ounce = 2 tablespoon

1 tablespoon = 3 teaspoons

1 teaspoon = 5 milliliters or 60 drops

1 gram = 1000 milligrams (mg) or 15.4 grains

two capsules = one teaspoon of tincture

two tablespoons tincture = one-half cup of infusion or decoction.